Preventing
CHRONIC DISEASES
a vital investment

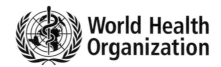
World Health
Organization

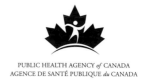

PUBLIC HEALTH AGENCY *of* CANADA
AGENCE DE SANTÉ PUBLIQUE *du* CANADA

WHO Library Cataloguing-in-Publication Data

World Health Organization.
Preventing chronic diseases : a vital investment : WHO global report.
1.Chronic disease – therapy 2.Investments 3.Evidence-based medicine 4.Public policy 5.Intersectoral cooperation I.Title.
ISBN 92 4 156300 1   (NLM classification: WT 500)

This report was produced under the overall direction of Catherine Le Galès-Camus (Assistant Director-General, Noncommunicable Diseases and Mental Health), Robert Beaglehole (Editor-in-Chief) and JoAnne Epping-Jordan (Managing Editor). The core contributors were Dele Abegunde, Robert Beaglehole, Stéfanie Durivage, JoAnne Epping-Jordan, Colin Mathers, Bakuti Shengelia, Kate Strong, Colin Tukuitonga and Nigel Unwin.

Guidance was offered throughout the production of the report by an Advisory Group: Catherine Le Galès-Camus, Andres de Francisco, Stephen Matlin, Jane McElligott, Christine McNab, Isabel Mortara, Margaret Peden, Thomson Prentice, Laura Sminkey, Ian Smith, Nigel Unwin and Janet Voûte.

External expert review was provided by: Olusoji Adeyi, Julien Bogousslavsky, Debbie Bradshaw, Jonathan Betz Brown, Robert Burton, Catherine Coleman, Ronald Dahl, Michael Engelgau, Majid Ezzati, Valentin Fuster, Pablo Gottret, Kei Kawabata, Steven Leeder, Pierre Lefèbvre, Karen Lock, James Mann, Mario Maranhão, Stephen Matlin, Martin McKee, Isabel Mortara, Thomas Pearson, Maryse Pierre-Louis, G. N. V. Ramana, Anthony Rodgers, Inés Salas, George Schieber, Linda Siminerio, Colin Sindall, Krisela Steyn, Boyd Swinburn, Michael Thiede, Theo Vos, Janet Voûte, Derek Yach and Ping Zhang.

Valuable input, help and advice were received from policy advisers to the Director-General and many technical staff at WHO Geneva, regional directors and members of their staff, WHO country representatives and country office staff.

Contributions were received from the following WHO regional and country office staff: Mohamed Amri, Alberto Barcèlo, Robert Burton, Luis Gerardo Castellanos, Lucimar Coser-Cannon, Niklas Danielsson, Jill Farrington, Antonio Filipé Jr, Gauden Galea, Josefa Ippolito-Shepherd, Oussama Khatib, Jerzy Leowski, Silvana Luciani, Gudjon Magnússon, Sylvia Robles, Aushra Shatchkute, Marc Suhrcke, Cristobal Tunon, Cherian Varghese and Yanwei Wu.

Report development and production were coordinated by Robert Beaglehole, JoAnne Epping-Jordan, Stéfanie Durivage, Amanda Marlin, Karen McCaffrey, Alexandra Munro, Caroline Savitzky, Kristin Thompson, with the administrative and secretarial support of Elmira Adenova, Virgie Largado-Ferri and Rachel Pedersen.

The report was edited by Leo Vita-Finzi. Translation coordination was provided by Peter McCarey. The web site and other electronic media were organized by Elmira Adenova, Catherine Needham and Andy Pattison. Proofreading was by Barbara Campanini. The index was prepared by Kathleen Lyle. Distribution was organized by Maryvonne Grisetti.

Design: Reda Sadki

Layout: Steve Ewart, Reda Sadki

Figures: Steve Ewart, Christophe Grangier

Photography: Chris De Bode, Panos Pictures, United Kingdom

Printing coordination: Robert Constandse, Raphaël Crettaz

Printed in Switzerland

More information about this publication and about chronic disease prevention and control can be obtained from:
Department of Chronic Diseases and Health Promotion
World Health Organization
CH-1211 Geneva 27, Switzerland
E-mail: chronicdiseases@who.int
Web site: http://www.who.int/chp/chronic_disease_report/en/

The production of this publication was made possible through the generous financial support of the Government of Canada, the Government of Norway and the Government of the United Kingdom.

CONTENTS

face to face
WITH **CHRONIC DISEASE**

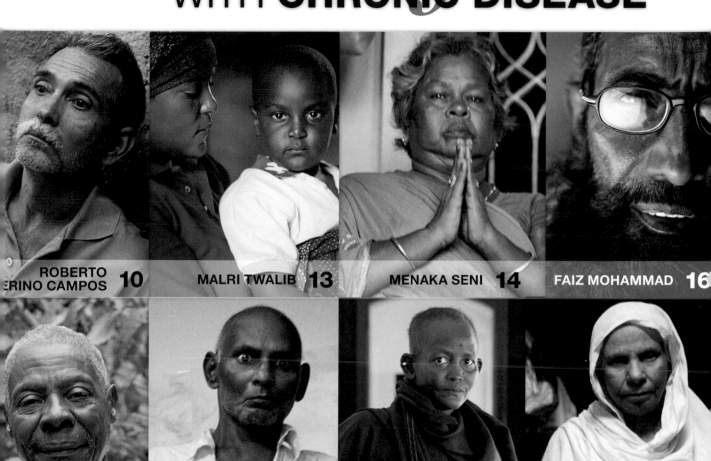

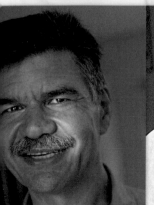
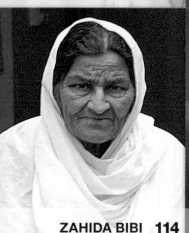
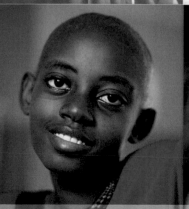
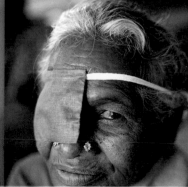

THE COST C
IS CLEAR AND

"The lives of far too many people in the world are being blighted and cut short by chronic diseases such as heart disease, stroke, cancer, chronic respiratory diseases and diabetes."

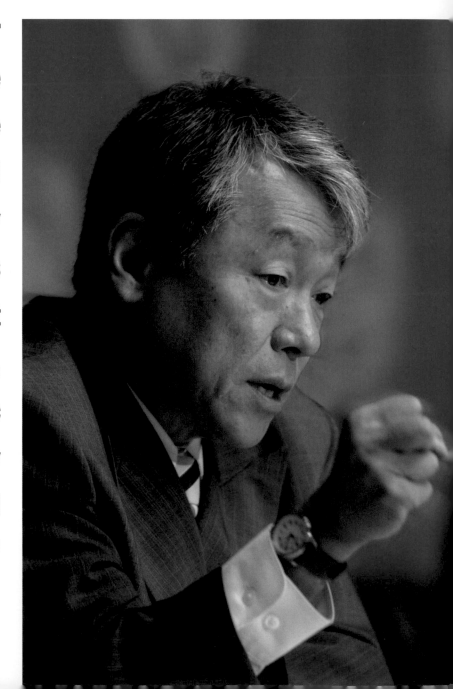

INACTION UNACCEPTABLE

The lives of far too many people in the world are being blighted and cut short by chronic diseases such as heart disease, stroke, cancer, chronic respiratory diseases and diabetes. This is no longer only happening in high income countries. Four out of five chronic disease deaths today are in low and middle income countries. People in these countries tend to develop diseases at younger ages, suffer longer – often with preventable complications – and die sooner than those in high income countries.

Globally, of the 58 million deaths in 2005, approximately 35 million will be as a result of chronic diseases. They are currently the major cause of death among adults in almost all countries and the toll is projected to increase by a further 17% in the next 10 years. At the same time, child overweight and obesity are increasing worldwide, and incidence of type 2 diabetes is growing.

This is a very serious situation, both for public health and for the societies and economies affected. Until recently, the impact and profile of chronic disease has generally been insufficiently appreciated. This ground-breaking report presents the most recent data, making clear the actual scale and severity of the problem and the urgent need for action.

The means of preventing and controlling most chronic diseases are already well-established. It is vital that countries review and implement the interventions described, taking a comprehensive and integrated public health approach.

The cost of inaction is clear and unacceptable. Through investing in vigorous and well-targeted prevention and control now, there is a real opportunity to make significant progress and improve the lives of populations across the globe.

LEE Jong-wook
Director-General, World Health Organization

A RESPONSIBILITY TO SAFEGUARD HEALTH

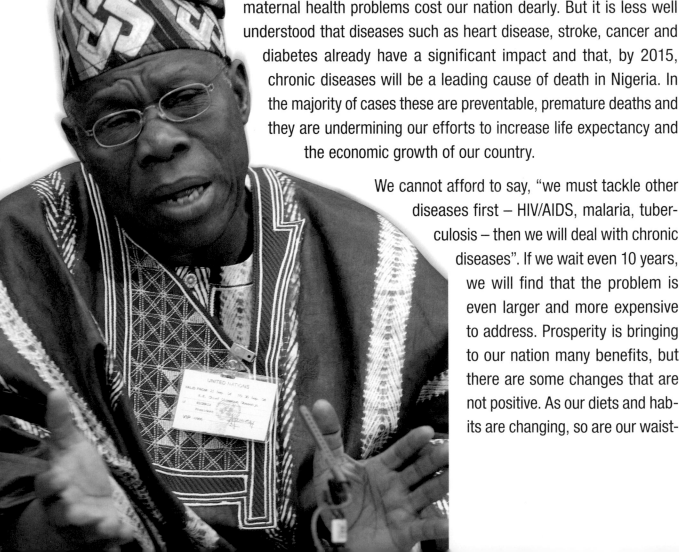

As the leader of the most populous country in Africa, I carry a responsibility to safeguard and improve the health, security and prosperity of Nigeria's people. I have looked at the facts contained in this report and I can see that to meet these challenges I will have to address chronic diseases.

It is widely known that HIV/AIDS, malaria, tuberculosis and child and maternal health problems cost our nation dearly. But it is less well understood that diseases such as heart disease, stroke, cancer and diabetes already have a significant impact and that, by 2015, chronic diseases will be a leading cause of death in Nigeria. In the majority of cases these are preventable, premature deaths and they are undermining our efforts to increase life expectancy and the economic growth of our country.

We cannot afford to say, "we must tackle other diseases first – HIV/AIDS, malaria, tuberculosis – then we will deal with chronic diseases". If we wait even 10 years, we will find that the problem is even larger and more expensive to address. Prosperity is bringing to our nation many benefits, but there are some changes that are not positive. As our diets and habits are changing, so are our waistlines. Already, more than 35% of women in Nigeria are overweight; by 2010 this number will rise to 44%.

We do not need to say, "we are a poor nation, we cannot afford to deal with chronic diseases". As this report points out, there are low-cost, effective measures that any country can take. We must tackle this problem step by step and we must start now.

Governments have a responsibility to support their citizens in their pursuit of a healthy, long life. It is not enough to say, "we have told them not to smoke, we have told them to eat fruit and vegetables, we have told them to take regular exercise". We must create communities, schools, workplaces and markets that make these healthy choices possible.

I believe, and the evidence supports me, that there are clear links between health, economic development and poverty alleviation. If my government and I are to build a strong Nigeria, and if my brothers and sisters throughout Africa are to create a strong continent, then we must include chronic diseases in our thinking. Let us use this report as a wake-up call. If we take action now, it could be that the predictions outlined in these analyses never come true.

I will join with the World Health Organization to implement the changes necessary in Nigeria, in the hope that we, too, can contribute towards achieving the global goal of reducing chronic disease death rates by 2% per year over the next 10 years, saving 36 million lives by 2015. That would be the most important inheritance we could pass on to our children.

Olusegun OBASANJO
President, Federal Republic of Nigeria

India

FACING CHRONIC DISEASES WITH ENERGY AND FOCUS

In India, as in many developing countries, public health advocacy to date has been mainly devoted to infectious diseases. However, we now have major public health issues due to chronic diseases that need to be addressed with equal energy and focus.

This World Health Organization report, *Preventing chronic diseases: a vital investment,* is of relevance to me, as Indian Minister for Health, as my country tackles the increasing number of issues relating to chronic disease. The scale of the problem we face is clear with the projected number of deaths attributable to

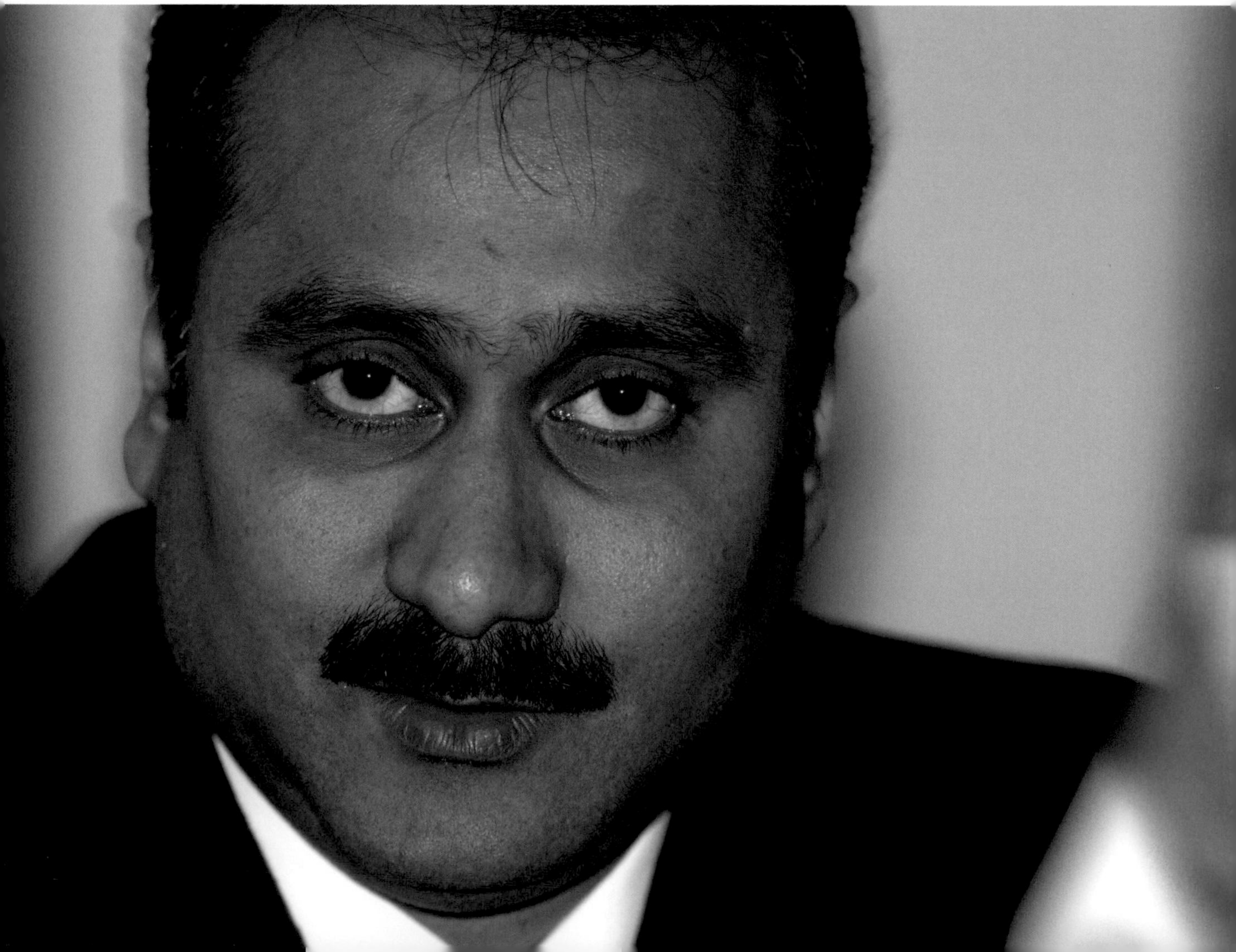

chronic diseases rising from 3.78 million in 1990 (40.4% of all deaths) to an expected 7.63 million in 2020 (66.7% of all deaths).

A number of my fellow citizens are featured within this report, as *Faces of Chronic Disease*. You will read about K. Sridhar Reddy, who, like a huge proportion of Indians, consumed tobacco and battled both serious cancer and associated financial debts. His story is all too familiar in a country which is the world's second largest producer, as well as consumer, of tobacco, where we consequently

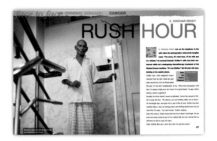

experience huge rates of cancer, including the largest numbers of oral cancer in the world. This costs the country dearly, for the individuals affected, but also in terms of treatment costs for tobacco-related diseases, estimated at US$ 7.2 billion just for the year 2002–2003.

Stories of hope include Menaka Seni, who faced potential tragedy when she suffered a heart attack. However, this proved to be the wake-up call she needed and she is now changing her health behaviour to tackle the weight and high blood pressure that have contributed to her heart disease and diabetes. Her diabetes problem is all too common in India, where we are at the top of the

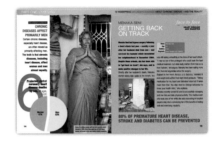

global league table for the number of people with the disease – an estimated 19.3 million in 1995, projected to rise to 57.2 million by 2025.

Some of the strategies for battling chronic disease have already been put in place. A National Cancer Control Programme, initiated in 1975, has established 13 cancer registries and increased the capacity for therapy. A comprehensive law for tobacco control was enacted in 2003. An integrated national programme for the prevention and control of cardiovascular diseases and diabetes is under development. But all these need to be scaled up. Additionally, we need to initiate comprehensive action to promote healthy diet and physical activity; and health services need to be reoriented to accommodate the needs of chronic disease prevention and control.

I believe that, if existing interventions are used together as a part of a comprehensive integrated approach, the global goal for preventing chronic disease can indeed be achieved and millions of lives saved. All segments of the society must unite across the world to provide a global thrust to counter this global threat. Governments must work together with the private sector and civil society to make this happen. This is a brighter future we can dedicate to children all around the world.

Dr Anbumani RAMADOSS
Minister of Health & Family Welfare, Government of India

People's Republic of China

A LONG-TERM INVESTMENT
IN THE FUTURE OF OUR CHILDREN

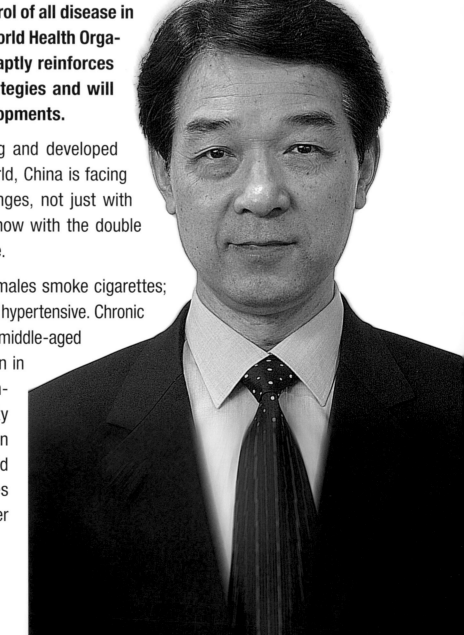

As the Vice-Minister for Health responsible for the prevention and control of all disease in China, I welcome this World Health Organization report, which aptly reinforces our current action strategies and will help guide future developments.

Like so many developing and developed countries around the world, China is facing significant health challenges, not just with infectious diseases but now with the double burden of chronic disease.

300 million of our adult males smoke cigarettes; 160 million adults are now hypertensive. Chronic disease death rates in our middle-aged population are higher than in some high income countries. We have an obesity epidemic, with more than 20% of our 7–17 year old children in urban centres tipping the scales as either overweight or obese.

These risk factors will cause an unacceptable number of people to die prematurely and often after years of needless suffering and disability, and tragically, so many who have recently escaped poverty will be plunged back, due to the burden of health care costs. This situation is especially tragic considering that at least 80% of all heart disease, stroke and diabetes are preventable.

And our global economies will also suffer severe consequences from societies battling chronic diseases. We can measure the loss of income to the Chinese economy alone at a staggering US$ 550 billion over the next 10 years, due to the effects of just heart disease, stroke and diabetes.

In response to these facts, the Ministry of Health of China, with the support of WHO, has been developing the first medium and long-term high level national plan for chronic disease control and prevention (2005–2015). In 2002 we established the National Centre for Chronic and Non-communicable Disease Control and Prevention (NCNCD), to be responsible for surveillance and population-based interventions. Currently a national chronic disease control network is being built to comprehensively survey our population. This is the type of comprehensive and integrated action that will achieve success in combating chronic diseases.

These programmes represent a long-term investment in our future, in the future of our children. We are committed to implementing the strategies outlined in this report to effectively prevent chronic disease and urge the same scale of commitment from others.

WANG Longde
Vice-Minister of Health, the People's Republic of China

WHAT'S INSIDE

This WHO global report:

» makes the case for urgent action to halt and turn back the growing threat of chronic diseases;

» presents a state-of-the-art guide to effective and feasible interventions;

» provides practical suggestions for how countries can implement these interventions to respond successfully to the growing epidemics.

The report focuses on the prevention of the major chronic conditions, primarily:

» heart disease and stroke (cardiovascular diseases);

» cancer;

» asthma and chronic obstructive pulmonary disease (chronic respiratory diseases);

» diabetes.

Other chronic diseases are highlighted selectively.

Global and regional information is presented. In addition to WHO regional groupings, World Bank income groupings are used. Based on its 2001 gross national income (GNI) per capita, each country is classified as follows:

» low income country: GNI per capita of US$ 745 or less;

» lower middle income country: GNI per capita of US$ 746–2975;

» upper middle income country: GNI per capita of US$ 2976–9205;

» high income country: GNI per capita of US$ 9206 or more.[1]

Nine selected countries are also featured in the report. The nine were chosen on the basis of the size of their chronic disease burden, quality and reliability of available data, and lessons learnt from previous prevention and control experiences.

» Brazil (upper middle income country)

» Canada (high income country)

» China (lower middle income country)

» India (low income country)

» Nigeria (low income country)

» Pakistan (low income country)

» Russian Federation (lower middle income country)

» United Kingdom (high income country)

» United Republic of Tanzania (low income country)

Other countries are highlighted selectively for examples of success and best practice.

[1] Categories for this report were based on the income categories published in *World development indicators 2003*. Washington, DC, World Bank, 2003.

Part One summarizes the report's main messages.

Part Two provides an overview of the risk factors and burden of chronic disease globally, regionally, and in selected countries. It also describes the links between chronic diseases and poverty, details the economic impact of chronic diseases, and presents a global goal for prevention of chronic diseases.

Part Three presents evidence-based interventions for the prevention and control of chronic diseases. Effective interventions for both the whole population and individuals are reviewed.

Part Four outlines a public health approach that governments can follow to formulate and implement an effective chronic disease policy. This part also describes the positive roles that the private sector and civil society can play.

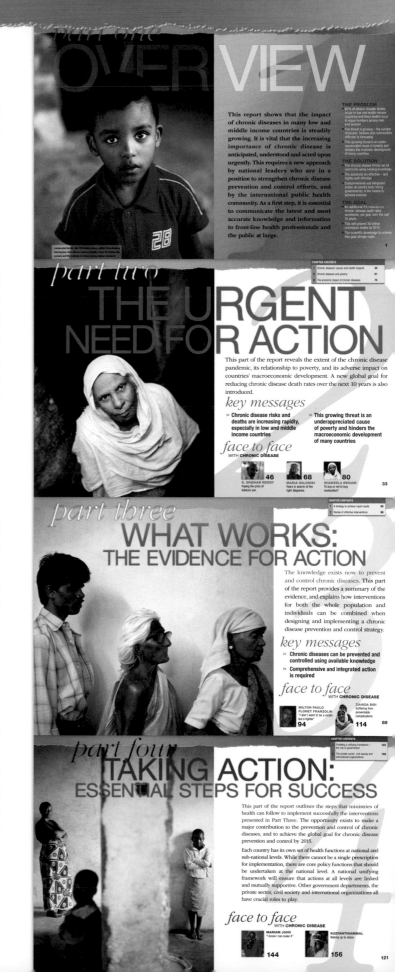

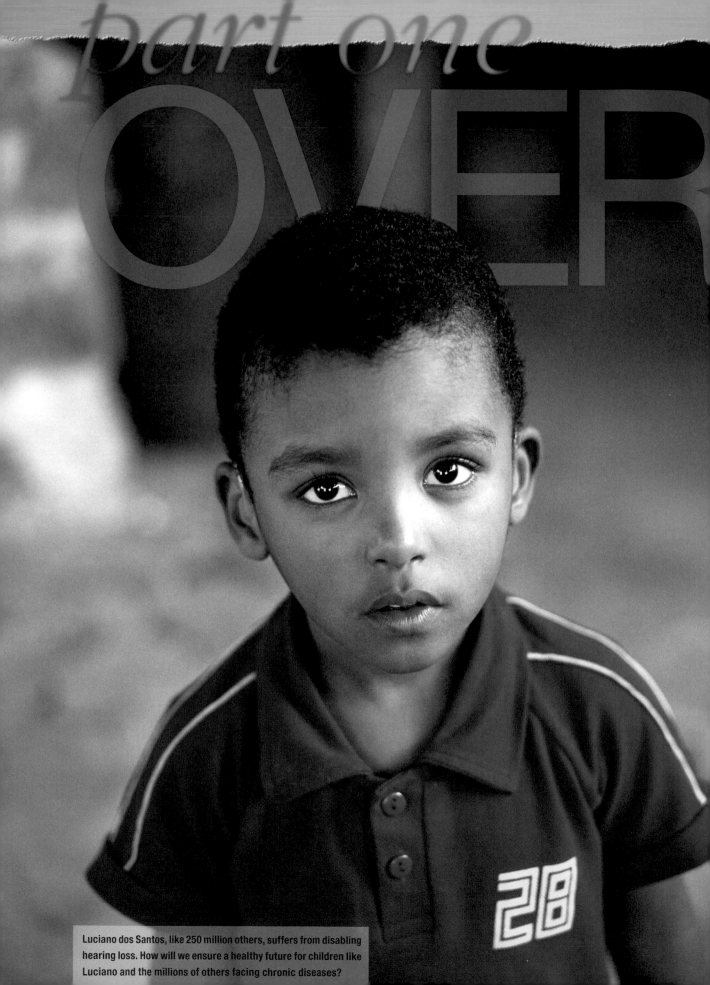

Luciano dos Santos, like 250 million others, suffers from disabling hearing loss. How will we ensure a healthy future for children like Luciano and the millions of others facing chronic diseases?

VIEW

This report shows that the impact of chronic diseases in many low and middle income countries is steadily growing. It is vital that the increasing importance of chronic disease is anticipated, understood and acted upon urgently. This requires a new approach by national leaders who are in a position to strengthen chronic disease prevention and control efforts, and by the international public health community. As a first step, it is essential to communicate the latest and most accurate knowledge and information to front-line health professionals and the public at large.

THE PROBLEM

» 80% of chronic disease deaths occur in low and middle income countries and these deaths occur in equal numbers among men and women

» The threat is growing – the number of people, families and communities afflicted is increasing

» This growing threat is an under-appreciated cause of poverty and hinders the economic development of many countries

THE SOLUTION

» The chronic disease threat can be overcome using existing knowledge

» The solutions are effective – and highly cost-effective

» Comprehensive and integrated action at country level, led by governments, is the means to achieve success

THE GOAL

» An additional 2% reduction in chronic disease death rates worldwide, per year, over the next 10 years

» This will prevent 36 million premature deaths by 2015

» The scientific knowledge to achieve this goal already exists

CHRONIC DISEASES ARE T
IN ALMOST ALL COUNTRIES

Chronic diseases include heart disease, stroke, cancer, chronic respiratory diseases and diabetes. Visual impairment and blindness, hearing impairment and deafness, oral diseases and genetic disorders are other chronic conditions that account for a substantial portion of the global burden of disease.

From a projected total of 58 million deaths from all causes in 2005,[1] it is estimated that chronic diseases will account for 35 million, which is double the number of deaths from all infectious diseases (including HIV/AIDS, tuberculosis and malaria), maternal and perinatal conditions, and nutritional deficiencies combined.

[1] The data presented in this overview were estimated by WHO using standard methods to maximize cross-country comparability. They are not necessarily the official statistics of Member States.

Projected

all ages, 200

35 000 000
people will die from
chronic diseases
in 2005

2 830 000 deaths

HIV/AIDS

1 607 000 deaths

Tuberculo

60%

MAJOR CAUSE OF DEATH

al deaths by cause,

883 000 deaths

17 528 000 deaths

7 586 000 deaths

4 057 000 deaths

1 125 000 deaths

Malaria

Cardiovascular
diseases

Cancer

Chronic
respiratory
diseases

Diabetes

f all deaths are due
o chronic diseases

3

THE POOREST COUNTRIES
ARE THE WORST AFFECTED

Only 20% of chronic disease deaths occur in high income countries – while 80% occur in low and middle income countries, where most of the world's population lives. As this report will show, even least developed countries such as the United Republic of Tanzania are not immune to the growing problem.

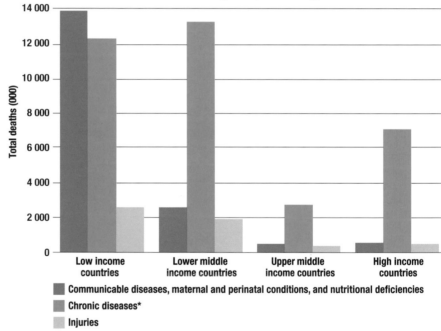

Projected deaths by major cause and World Bank income group, all ages, 2005

Total deaths (000)

14 000
12 000
10 000
8 000
6 000
4 000
2 000
0

Low income countries | Lower middle income countries | Upper middle income countries | High income countries

■ Communicable diseases, maternal and perinatal conditions, and nutritional deficiencies
■ Chronic diseases*
■ Injuries

* Chronic diseases include cardiovascular diseases, cancers, chronic respiratory disorders, diabetes, neuropsychiatric and sense organ disorders, musculoskeletal and oral disorders, digestive diseases, genito-urinary diseases, congenital abnormalities and skin diseases.

80% of chronic disease deaths occur in low and middle income countries

Projected foregone national income
due to heart disease, stroke and diabetes
in selected countries, 2005–2015

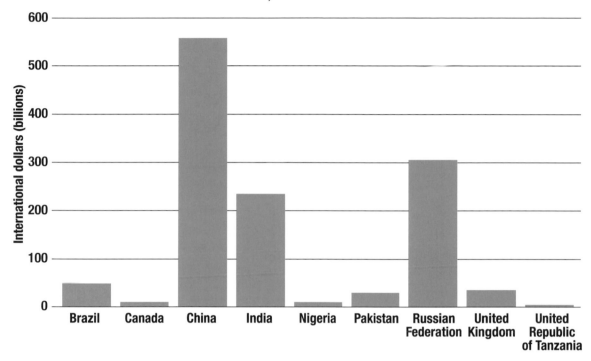

THE PROBLEM HAS SERIOUS IMPACT

The burden of chronic disease:

» has major adverse effects on the quality of life of affected individuals;

» causes premature death;

» creates large adverse – and underappreciated – economic effects on families, communities and societies in general.

$558 billion

The estimated amount China will forego in national income over the next 10 years as a result of premature deaths caused by heart disease, stroke and diabetes

THE RISK FACTORS ARE WIDESPREAD

Common, modifiable risk factors underlie the major chronic diseases. These risk factors explain the vast majority of chronic disease deaths at all ages, in men and women, and in all parts of the world. They include:

» unhealthy diet;

» physical inactivity;

» tobacco use.

Each year at least:

» 4.9 million people die as a result of tobacco use;

» 2.6 million people die as a result of being overweight or obese;

» 4.4 million people die as a result of raised total cholesterol levels;

» 7.1 million people die as a result of raised blood pressure.

THE THREAT IS GROWING

Deaths from infectious diseases, maternal and perinatal conditions, and nutritional deficiencies combined are projected to decline by 3% over the next 10 years. In the same period, deaths due to chronic diseases are projected to increase by 17%.

This means that of the projected 64 million people who will die in 2015, 41 million will die of a chronic disease – unless urgent action is taken.

1 000 000 000
people are overweight

THE GLOBAL RESPONSE IS
INADEQUATE

Despite global successes, such as the WHO Framework Convention on Tobacco Control, the first legal instrument designed to reduce tobacco-related deaths and disease around the world, chronic diseases have generally been neglected in international health and development work.

Furthermore, chronic diseases – the major cause of adult illness and death in all regions of the world – have not been included within the global Millennium Development Goal (MDG) targets; although as a recent WHO publication on health and the MDGs has recognized, there is scope for doing so within Goal 6 (Combat HIV/AIDS, malaria and other diseases). Health more broadly, including chronic disease prevention, contributes to poverty reduction and hence Goal 1 (Eradicate extreme poverty and hunger).[1] In response to their needs, several countries have already adapted their MDG targets and indicators to include chronic diseases and/or their risk factors; a selection of these countries is featured in Part Two.

This report will demonstrate that chronic diseases hinder economic growth and reduce the development potential of countries, and this is especially true for countries experiencing rapid economic growth, such as China and India. However, it is important that prevention is addressed within the context of international health and development work even in least developed countries such as the United Republic of Tanzania, which are already undergoing an upsurge in chronic disease risks and deaths.

[1] *Health and the Millennium Development Goals.* Geneva, World Health Organization, 2005.

388 000 000
people will die in the next 10 years of a chronic disease

10 WIDESPREAD MI:

ABOUT CHRONIC DISEASE – AND THE REALITY

Several misunderstandings have contributed to the neglect of chronic disease. Notions that chronic diseases are a distant threat and are less important and serious than some infectious diseases can be dispelled by the strongest evidence. Ten of the most common misunderstandings are presented below.

Projected global distribution of chronic disease deaths
by World Bank income group, all ages, 2005

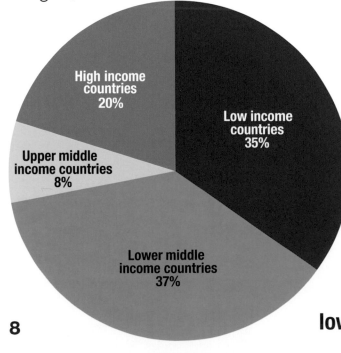

High income countries
20%

Low income countries
35%

Upper middle income countries
8%

Lower middle income countries
37%

8

MISUNDERSTANDING CHRONIC DISEASES MAINLY AFFECT HIGH INCOME COUNTRIES

Whereas the common notion is that chronic diseases mainly affect high income countries, the reality is that **four out of five chronic disease deaths are in low and middle income countries.**

Projected death rates by specific cause
for selected countries, all ages, 2005

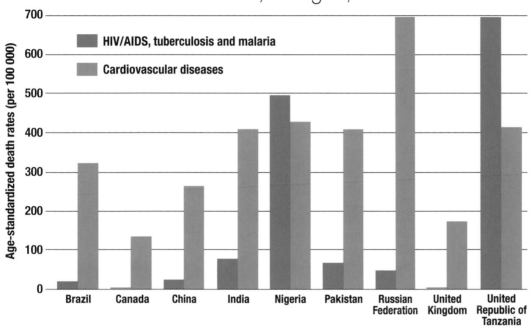

MISUNDERSTANDING LOW AND MIDDLE INCOME
COUNTRIES SHOULD CONTROL INFECTIOUS DISEASES
BEFORE CHRONIC DISEASES

Many people believe that low and middle income countries should control infectious diseases before they tackle chronic diseases. In reality, **low and middle income countries are at the centre of both old and new public health challenges.** While they continue to deal with the problems of infectious diseases, they are in many cases experiencing a rapid upsurge in chronic disease risk factors and deaths, especially in urban settings. These risk levels foretell a devastating future burden of chronic diseases in these countries.

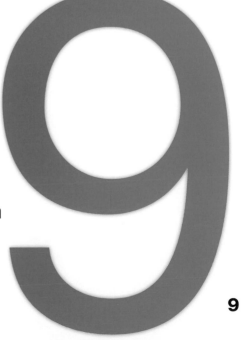

9

MISUNDERSTANDING
CHRONIC DISEASES MAINLY AFFECT RICH PEOPLE

Many people think that chronic diseases mainly affect rich people. The truth is that in all but the least developed countries of the world, poor people are much more likely than the wealthy to develop chronic diseases, and everywhere are more likely to die as a result. Moreover, chronic diseases cause substantial financial burden, and can push individuals and households into poverty.

ROBERTO SEVERINO CAMPOS
FACING ILLNESS AND DEEPENING POVERTY

Roberto Severino Campos lives in a shanty town in the outskirts of São Paulo with his seven children and 16 grandchildren. Roberto never paid attention to his high blood pressure, nor to his drinking and smoking habits. "He was so stubborn," his 31-year-old daughter Noemia recalls, "that we couldn't talk about his health".

Roberto had his first stroke six years ago at the age of 46 – it paralysed his legs. He then lost his ability to speak after two consecutive strokes four years later. Roberto used to work as a public transport agent, but now depends entirely on his family to survive.

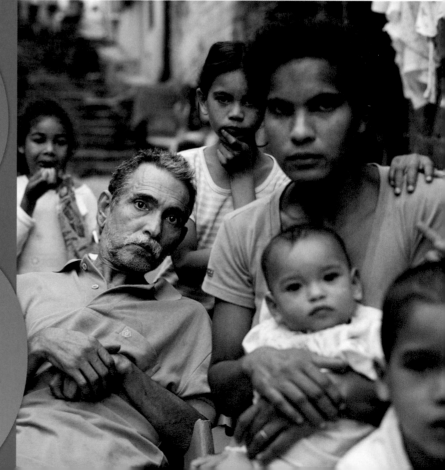

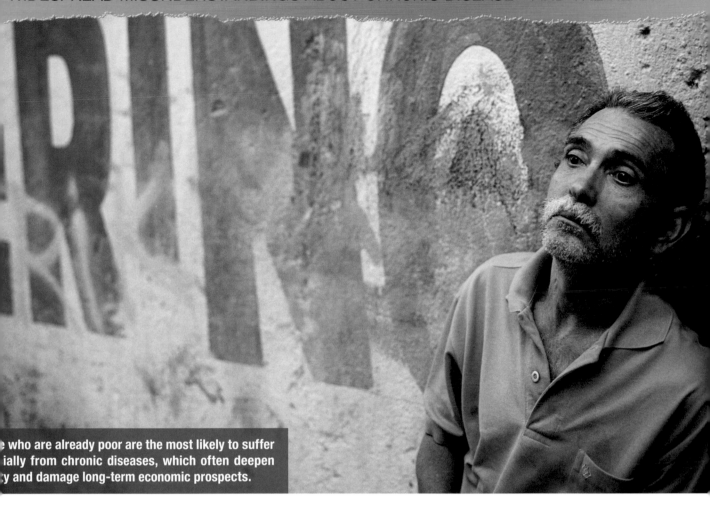

e who are already poor are the most likely to suffer ially from chronic diseases, which often deepen y and damage long-term economic prospects.

BRAZIL

face to face
WITH CHRONIC DISEASE: STROKE

Name	Roberto Severino Campos
Age	52
Country	Brazil
Diagnosis	Stroke

Since Roberto's first stroke, his wife has been working long hours as a cleaner to earn money for the family. Their eldest son is also helping with expenses. Much of the family's income is used to buy the special diapers that Roberto needs. "Fortunately his medication and check-ups are free of charge but sometimes we just don't have the money for the bus to take us to the local medical centre," Noemia continues. But the burden is even greater: this family not only lost its breadwinner, but also a devoted father and grandfather, in whom each family member could confide.

Roberto is now trapped in his own body and always needs someone to feed him and see to his most basic needs. Noemia carries him in and out of the house so he can take a breath of air from time to time. "We all wish we could get him a wheelchair," she says.

Noemia and four of her brothers and sisters also suffer from high blood pressure.

MISUNDERSTANDING **CHRONIC DISEASES MAINLY AFFECT OLD PEOPLE**

Chronic diseases are often viewed as primarily affecting old people. We now know that **almost half of chronic disease deaths occur prematurely, in people under 70 years of age.** One quarter of all chronic disease deaths occur in people under 60 years of age.

In low and middle income countries, middle-aged adults are especially vulnerable to chronic disease. People in these countries tend to develop disease at younger ages, suffer longer – often with preventable complications – and die sooner than those in high income countries.

Childhood overweight and obesity is a rising global problem. About 22 million children aged under five years are overweight. In the United Kingdom, the prevalence of overweight in children aged two to

10 years rose from 23% to 28% between 1995 and 2003. In urban areas of China, overweight and obesity among children aged two to six years increased substantially from 1989 to 1997. Reports of type 2 diabetes in children and adolescents – previously unheard of – have begun to mount worldwide.

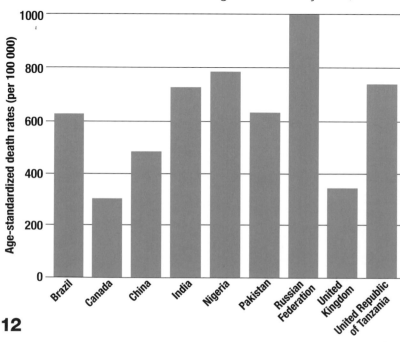

Projected chronic disease death rates
for selected countries, aged 30–69 years, 2005

MALRI TWALIB
THE NEXT GENERATION

MALRI TWALIB IS A FIVE-YEAR-OLD BOY living in a poor rural area of the Kilimanjaro District of the United Republic of Tanzania. Health workers from a nearby medical centre spotted his weight problem last year during a routine community outreach activity. The diagnosis was clear: childhood obesity.

Name	Malri Twalib
Age	5
Country	United Republic of Tanzania
Diagnosis	Obesity

One year later, Malri's health condition hasn't changed for the better and neither has his excessive consumption of porridge and animal fat. His fruit and vegetable intake also remains seriously insufficient – "it is just too hard to find reasonably priced products during the dry season, so I can't manage his diet," his mother Fadhila complains.

The community health workers who recently visited Malri for a follow-up also noticed that he was holding the same flat football as before – the word "Health" stamped on it couldn't pass unnoticed. Malri's neighbourhood is littered with sharp and rusted construction debris and the courtyard is too small for him to be able to play ball games. In fact, he rarely plays outside. "It is simply too hazardous. He could get hurt," his mother says.

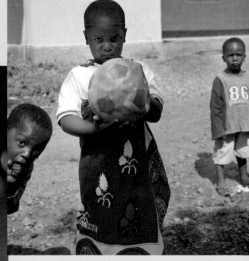

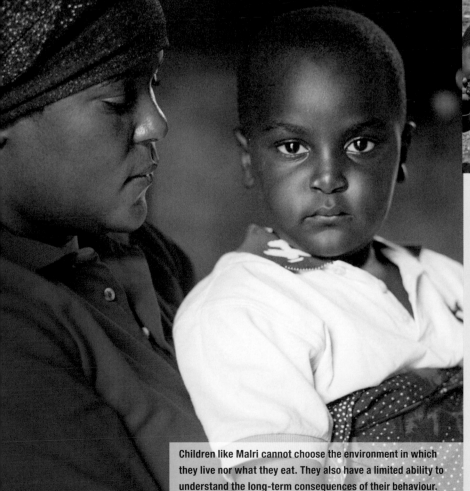

Fadhila, who is herself obese, believes that there are no risks attached to her son's obesity and that his weight will naturally go down one day. "Rounded forms run in the family and there's no history of chronic diseases, so why make a big fuss of all this," she argues with a smile on her face. In fact, Malri and Fadhila are at risk of developing a chronic disease as a result of their obesity.

Children like Malri cannot choose the environment in which they live nor what they eat. They also have a limited ability to understand the long-term consequences of their behaviour.

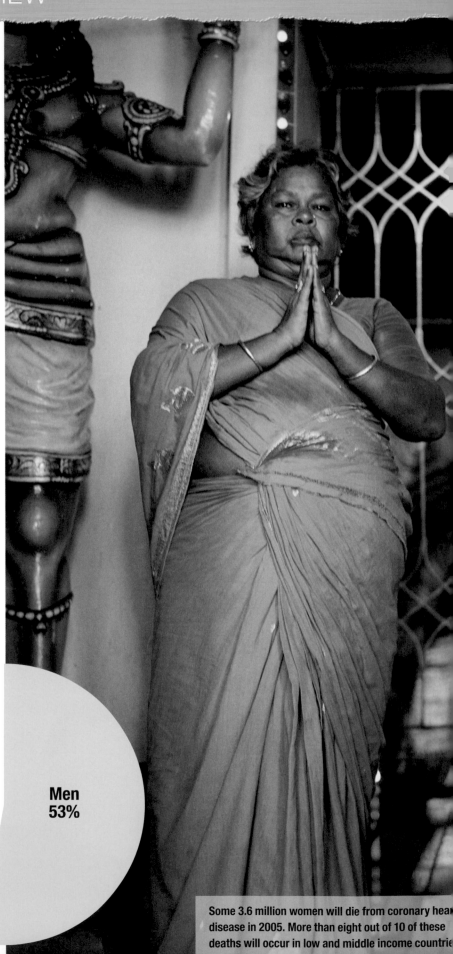

CHRONIC DISEASES AFFECT PRIMARILY MEN

Certain chronic diseases, especially heart disease, are often viewed as primarily affecting men. The truth is that **chronic diseases, including heart disease, affect women and men almost equally.**

Projected global coronary heart disease deaths by sex, all ages, 2005

Women
47%

Men
53%

14

Some 3.6 million women will die from coronary heart disease in 2005. More than eight out of 10 of these deaths will occur in low and middle income countries

MENAKA SENI
GETTING BACK ON TRACK

Menaka Seni had bypass surgery following a heart attack last year – exactly a year after her husband died from one – and survived the tsunami which devastated her neighbourhood in December 2004. Despite these ordeals, she has been able to "get back on track", she says, and to make positive changes to her life.

Shortly after her husband's death, Menaka started taking daily walks to the temple, but

Name	Menaka Seni
Age	60
Country	India
Diagnosis	Heart disease and diabetes

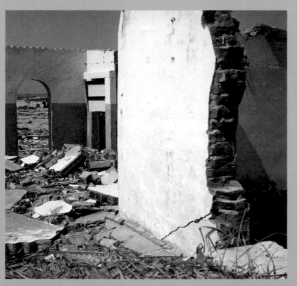

was still eating unhealthily at the time of her heart attack. "I may be one of the privileged who could seek the best medical treatment, but what really matters from now on is how I behave," she argues. Menaka has been eating more fish, fruit and vegetables since the surgery.

Related to her heart disease and diabetes, Menaka is overweight and suffers from high blood pressure. "Taking medication for my heart and diabetes helps but it takes more than that. You also need to change behaviour to lower your health risks," she explains.

Menaka recently turned 60 and is successfully managing both her diet and daily physical activity. The medical staff who took care of her while she was recovering in hospital played a key role in convincing her of the benefits of eating well and exercising regularly.

80% OF PREMATURE HEART DISEASE, STROKE AND DIABETES CAN BE PREVENTED

MISUNDERSTANDING
CHRONIC DISEASES ARE THE RESULT OF UNHEALTHY "LIFESTYLES"

Many people believe that if individuals develop chronic disease as a result of unhealthy "lifestyles", they have no one to blame but themselves. The truth is that **individual responsibility can have its full effect only where individuals have equitable access to a healthy life, and are supported to make healthy choices.** Governments have a crucial role to play in improving the health and well-being of populations, and in providing special protection for vulnerable groups.

This is especially true for children, who cannot choose the environment in which they live, their diet and their passive exposure to tobacco smoke. They also have a limited ability to understand the long-term consequences of their behaviour.

Poor people also have limited choices about the food they eat, their living conditions, and access to education and health care. Supporting healthy choices, especially for those who could not otherwise afford them, reduces risks and social inequalities.

PAKISTAN

FAIZ MOHAMMAD
"PEOPLE DON'T UNDERSTAND WHY I BECAME ILL"

Name	Faiz Mohammad
Age	48
Country	Pakistan
Diagnosis	Diabetes

FOR THE PAST 20 YEARS, Faiz Mohammad has been a victim of the misunderstandings surrounding his condition. He married two years after being diagnosed with diabetes, and remembers the difficulty he had in obtaining the blessing of his future parents-in-law. "They were quite reluctant to give their daughter to someone with diabetes. They didn't trust me. They thought I couldn't support a family," Faiz explains.

A hard-working livestock keeper and a father of three boys, Faiz considers that at 48 he's living a normal life. However, even after all this time, he still encounters all sorts of obstacles that he finds difficult to overcome. "People don't understand why I suddenly became ill. They think I have done something wrong and that I'm being punished."

Faiz himself has misunderstandings about his disease. He wrongly believes that diabetes is contagious and that he could transmit it sexually to his wife. "I'm afraid of contaminating her because people keep telling me that I will," he says.

Faiz has a check-up and buys insulin every two months at a local clinic. He claims that he is not receiving clear information about his disease and wishes he knew where to find answers to all his questions.

face to face
WITH **CHRONIC DISEASE:**
DIABETES

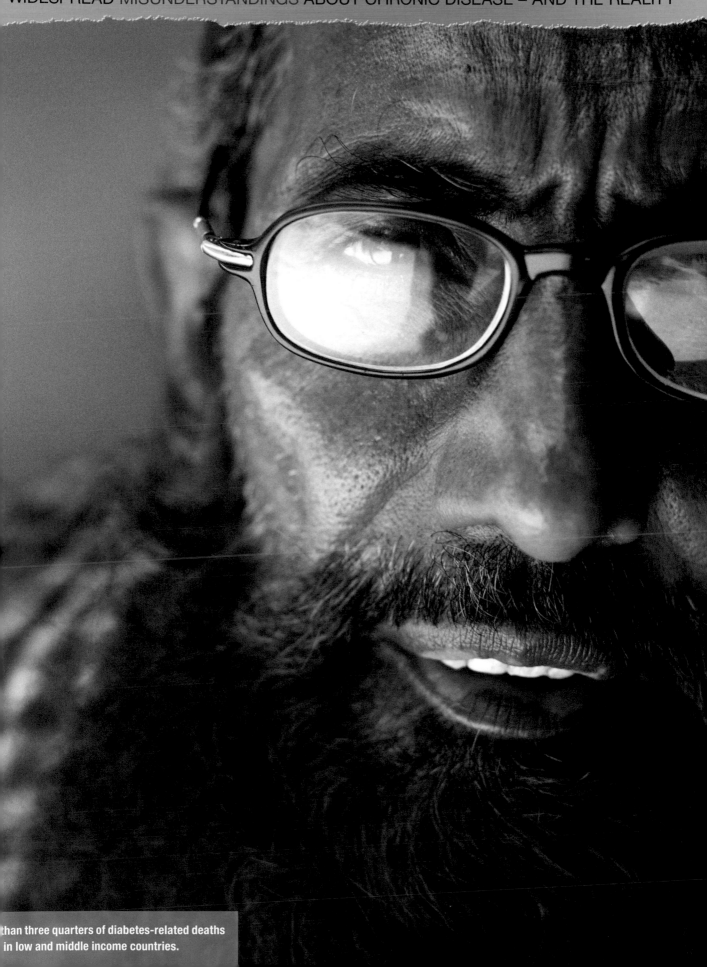

than three quarters of diabetes-related deaths in low and middle income countries.

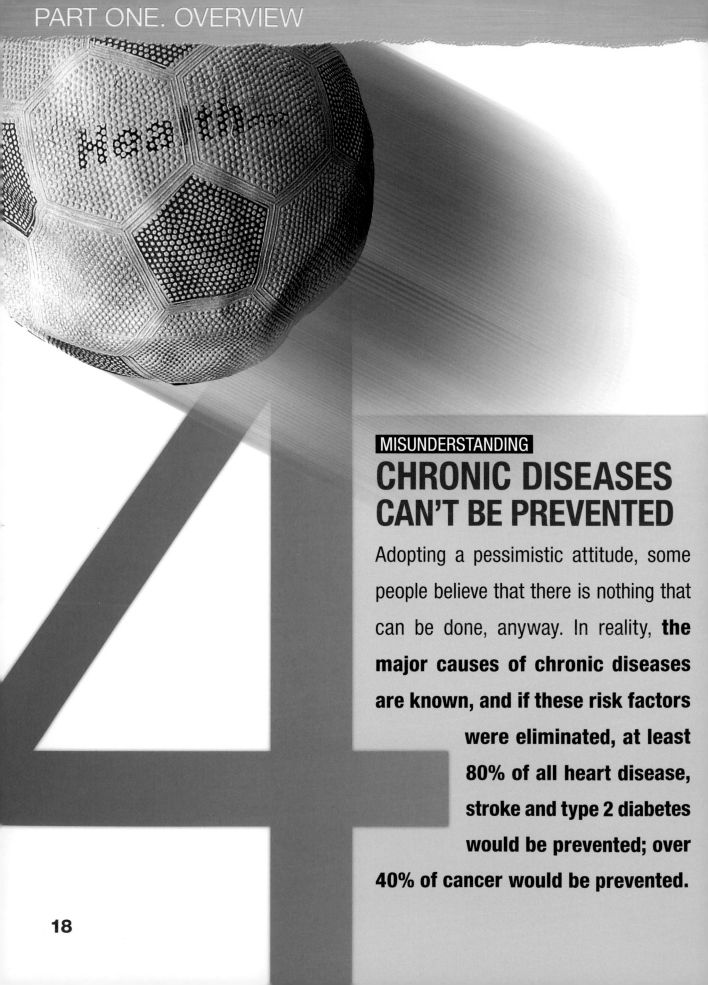

MISUNDERSTANDING

CHRONIC DISEASES CAN'T BE PREVENTED

Adopting a pessimistic attitude, some people believe that there is nothing that can be done, anyway. In reality, **the major causes of chronic diseases are known, and if these risk factors were eliminated, at least 80% of all heart disease, stroke and type 2 diabetes would be prevented; over 40% of cancer would be prevented.**

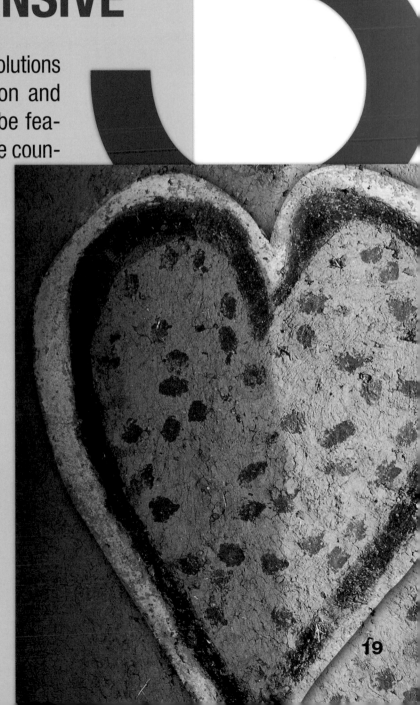

MISUNDERSTANDING

CHRONIC DISEASE
PREVENTION AND CONTROL
IS TOO EXPENSIVE

Some people believe that the solutions for chronic disease prevention and control are too expensive to be feasible for low and middle income countries. In reality, **a full range of chronic disease interventions are very cost-effective for all regions of the world, including sub-Saharan Africa. Many of these solutions are also inexpensive to implement.** The ideal components of a medication to prevent complications in people with heart disease, for example, are no longer covered by patent restrictions and could be produced for little more than one dollar a month.

HALF-TRUTHS Another set of misunderstandings arises from kernels of truth. In these cases, the kernels of truth are distorted to become sweeping statements that are not true. Because they are based on the truth, such half-truths are among the most ubiquitous and persistent misunderstandings. Two principal half-truths are refuted below.

HALF-TRUTH

"My grandfather smoked and was overweight – and he lived to 96"

In any population, there will be a certain number of people who do not demonstrate the typical patterns seen in the vast majority.

For chronic diseases, there are two major types:

» people with many chronic disease risk factors, who nonetheless live a healthy and long life;

» people with no or few chronic disease risk factors, who nonetheless develop chronic disease and/or die from complications at a young age.

These people undeniably exist, but they are rare. The vast majority of chronic disease can be traced back to the common risk factors, and can be prevented by eliminating these risks.

"HALF-TRUTH
Everyone has to die of something "

Certainly everyone has to die of something, but death does not need to be slow, painful, or premature.

Most chronic diseases do not result in sudden death. Rather, they are likely to cause people to become progressively ill and debilitated, especially if their illness is not managed correctly.

Death is inevitable, but a life of protracted ill-health is not. Chronic disease prevention and control helps people to live longer and healthier lives.

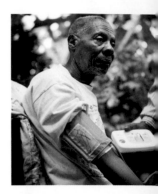

JONAS JUSTO KASSA
DYING SLOWLY, PAINFULLY AND PREMATURELY

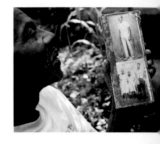

Name	Jonas Justo Kassa
Age	65
Country	United Republic of Tanzania
Diagnosis	Diabetes

BEFORE RETIRING as a mathematics teacher, Jonas Justo Kassa worked on his land after school hours and remembers that he was feeling very tired and constantly urinating. "I just assumed that I was working too hard, I wish I would have known better," he says with regret, 13 years down the road.

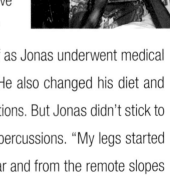

Despite these symptoms, Jonas waited several years before seeking help. "I first went to the traditional healer, but after months of taking the herb treatment he prescribed I wasn't feeling any better," he recalls. "So a friend drove me to the hospital – a 90 minute drive from here. I was diagnosed with diabetes in 1997."

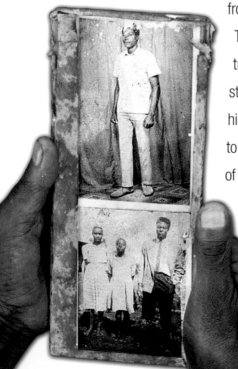

The next couple of years were an immense relief as Jonas underwent medical treatment to stabilize his blood glucose levels. He also changed his diet and stopped drinking under his doctor's recommendations. But Jonas didn't stick to his healthier ways for long, and it led to health repercussions. "My legs started to hurt in 2001. I couldn't measure my blood sugar and from the remote slopes of Kilimanjaro, it's difficult to reach a doctor," he explains.

The pain became much worse and complications that could have been avoided unfortunately appeared. Jonas had his right and left legs amputated in 2003 and 2004. "I now feel doomed and lonely. My friends have left me. I am of no use to them and my family anymore," he said with resignation before dying in his home, on 21 May 2005. Jonas was 65 years old.

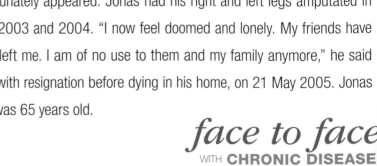

face to face
WITH **CHRONIC DISEASE:**
DIABETES

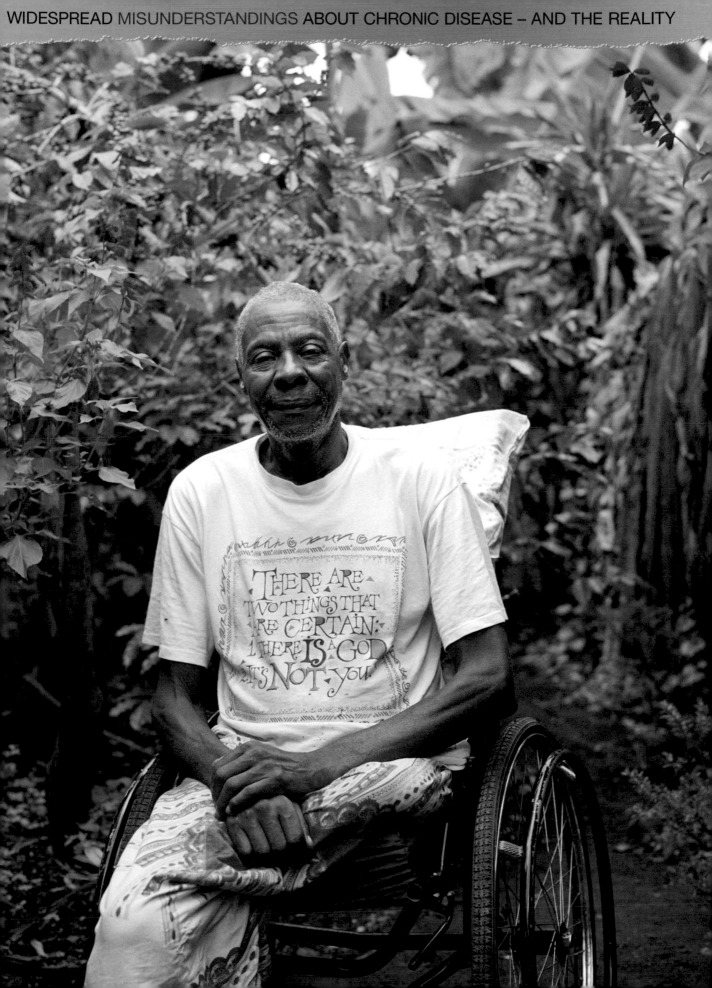

A VISION FOR REDUCING DEATHS

CHRONIC DISEASES CAN BE PREVENTED AND CONTROLLED

The rapid changes that threaten global health require a rapid response that must above all be forward-looking. The great epidemics of tomorrow are unlikely to resemble those that have previously swept the world, thanks to progress in infectious disease control. While the risk of outbreaks, such as a new influenza pandemic, will require constant vigilance, it is the "invisible" epidemics of heart disease, stroke, diabetes, cancer and other chronic diseases that for the foreseeable future will take the greatest toll in deaths and disability.

However, it is by no means a future without hope. For another of today's realities, equally well supported by the evidence, is that the means to prevent and treat chronic diseases, and to avoid millions of premature deaths and an immense burden of disability, already exist.

In several countries, the application of existing knowledge has led to major improvements in the life expectancy and quality of life of middle-aged and older people. For example, heart disease death rates have fallen by up to 70% in the last three decades in Australia, Canada, the United Kingdom and the United States. Middle income countries, such as Poland, have also been able to make substantial improvements in recent years. Such

THE FUTURE:
D IMPROVING LIVES

gains have been realized largely as a result of the implementation of comprehensive and integrated approaches that encompass interventions directed at both the whole population and individuals, and that focus on the common underlying risk factors, cutting across specific diseases.

The cumulative total of lives saved through these reductions is impressive. From 1970 to 2000, WHO has estimated that 14 million cardiovascular disease deaths were averted in the United States alone. The United Kingdom saved 3 million people during the same period.

Heart disease death rates among men aged 30 years or more, 1950–2002

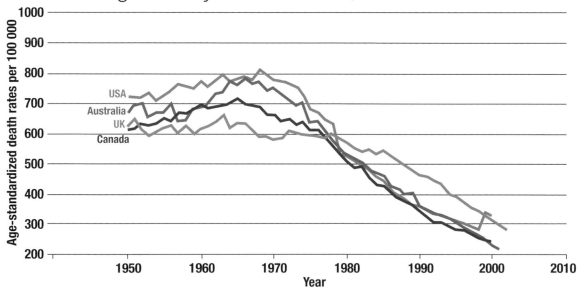

THE CHALLENGE IS NOW FOR OTHER COUNTRIES TO FOLLOW SUIT

2005 2006 2007 2008 2009 2010 2011 2012 2013 2014 2015

PREVENTING THE GLOBA

ENCOURAGED BY ACHIEVEMENTS in countries such as Australia, Canada, Poland, the United Kingdom and the United States, this report anticipates more such gains in the years ahead. But realistically, how much is possible by the year 2015? After carefully weighing all the available evidence, the report offers the health community a new global goal: to reduce death rates from all chronic diseases by 2% per year over and above existing trends during the next 10 years. This bold goal is thus in addition to the declines in age-specific death rates already projected for many chronic diseases, and would result in the prevention of 36 million chronic disease deaths by 2015, most of these being in low and middle income countries. Achievement of the global goal would also result in appreciable economic dividends for countries.

36 000 000 liv

RONIC DISEASES: GOAL FOR 2015

Every death averted is a bonus, but the goal contains an additional positive feature: almost half of these averted deaths would be in men and women under 70 years of age and almost nine out of 10 of these would be in low and middle income countries. Extending these lives for the benefit of the individuals concerned, their families and communities is in itself the worthiest of goals.

This global goal is ambitious and adventurous, but it is neither extravagant nor unrealistic. The means to achieve it, based on evidence and best practices from countries that have made improvements, are outlined in Parts Three and Four of this report.

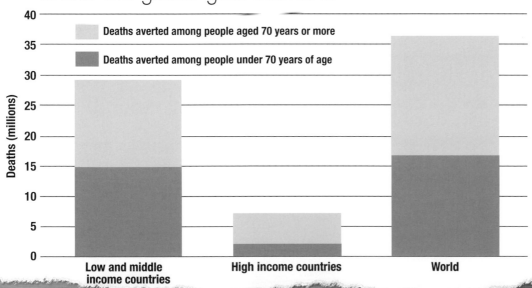

Estimated global deaths averted
under the global goal scenario

Legend:
- Deaths averted among people aged 70 years or more
- Deaths averted among people under 70 years of age

Y-axis: Deaths (millions) — 0, 5, 10, 15, 20, 25, 30, 35, 40

X-axis: Low and middle income countries | High income countries | World

can be saved

taking THE FIRS

Every country, regardless of the level of its resources, has the potential to make significant improvements in chronic disease prevention and control, and to take steps towards achieving the global goal. Resources are necessary, but a large amount can be achieved for little cost, and the benefits far outweigh the costs. Leadership is essential, and will have far more impact than simply adding capital to already overloaded health systems.

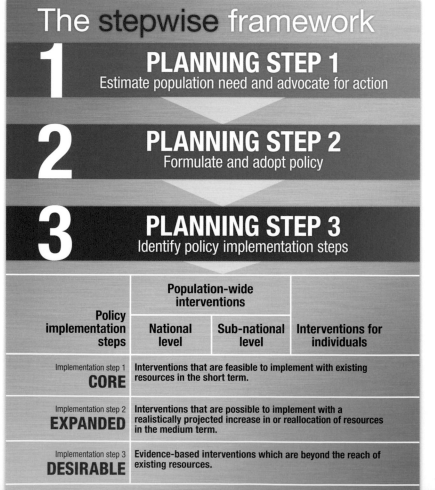

The stepwise framework

1 PLANNING STEP 1
Estimate population need and advocate for action

2 PLANNING STEP 2
Formulate and adopt policy

3 PLANNING STEP 3
Identify policy implementation steps

Policy implementation steps	Population-wide interventions		Interventions for individuals
	National level	Sub-national level	
Implementation step 1 **CORE**	Interventions that are feasible to implement with existing resources in the short term.		
Implementation step 2 **EXPANDED**	Interventions that are possible to implement with a realistically projected increase in or reallocation of resources in the medium term.		
Implementation step 3 **DESIRABLE**	Evidence-based interventions which are beyond the reach of existing resources.		

T STEPS

There is important work to be done in countries at all stages of development. In the poorest countries, many of which are experiencing upsurges in chronic disease risks, it is vital that supportive policies are in place to reduce risks and curb the epidemics before they take hold. In countries with established chronic disease problems, additional measures will be required, not only to prevent disease, but also to manage illness and disability.

Part Four of this report details the stepwise framework for implementing recommended measures. The framework offers a flexible and practical public health approach to assist ministries of health to balance diverse needs and priorities while implementing evidence-based interventions.

While there cannot be a "one size fits all" prescription for implementation – each country must consider a range of factors in establishing priorities – using the stepwise framework will make a major contribution to the prevention and control of chronic disease, and will assist countries in their efforts to achieve the global goal by 2015.

a final word

In many ways, we are the heirs of the choices that were made by previous generations: politicians, business leaders, financiers and ordinary people. Future generations will in turn be affected by the decisions that we make today.

Each of us has a choice: whether to continue with the status quo, or to take up the challenge and invest now in chronic disease prevention.

STATUS QUO

Without action, an estimated 388 million people will die from chronic diseases in the next 10 years. Many of these deaths will occur prematurely, affecting families, communities and countries.

The macroeconomic impact will be substantial. Countries such as China, India and the Russian Federation could forego between $200 billion and $550 billion in national income over the next 10 years as a result of heart disease, stroke and diabetes.

INVEST NOW

With **increased investment** in chronic disease prevention, as outlined in this report, it will be possible to **prevent 36 million premature deaths in the next 10 years**. Some 17 million of these prevented deaths would be among people under 70 years of age.

These averted deaths would also translate into **substantial gains in countries' economic growth**. For example, achievement of the global goal would result in an accumulated economic growth of $36 billion in China, $15 billion in India and $20 billion in the Russian Federation over the next 10 years.

The failure to use available knowledge about chronic disease prevention and control needlessly endangers future generations. There is simply no justification for chronic diseases to continue taking millions of lives prematurely each year while being overlooked on the health development agenda, when the understanding of how to prevent these deaths is available now.

Taking up the challenge of chronic disease prevention and control requires a certain amount of courage and ambition. The agenda is broad and bold, but the way forward is clear.

THE CAUSES ARE KNOWN.
THE WAY FORWARD IS CLEAR.
IT'S YOUR TURN TO TAKE ACTION.

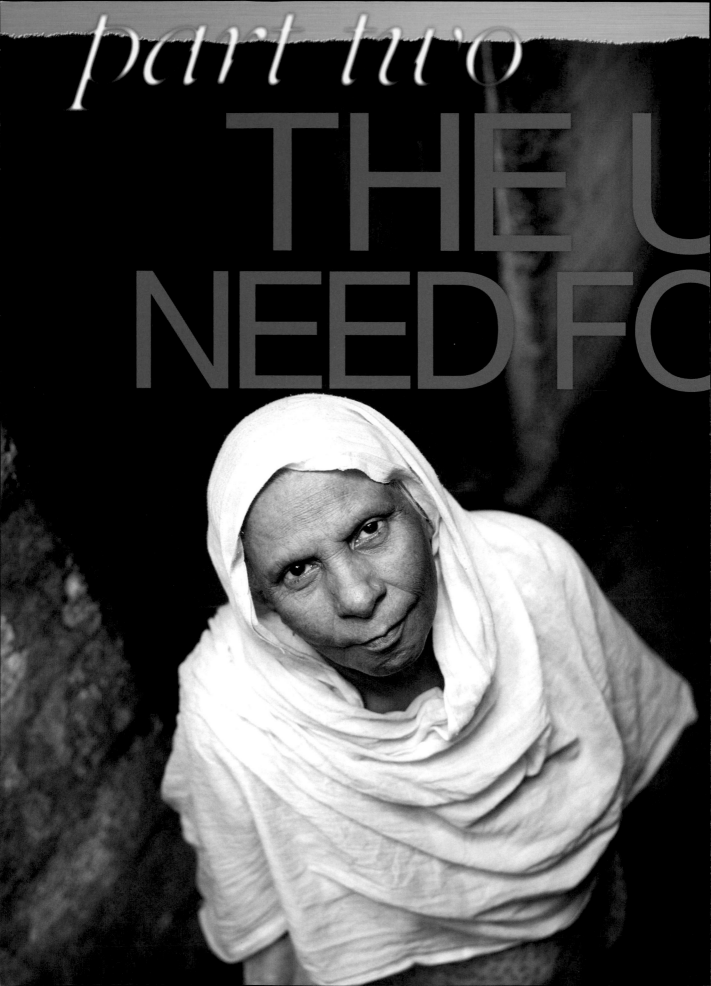

part two

THE U
NEED FO

RGENT
R ACTION

This part of the report reveals the extent of the chronic disease pandemic, its relationship to poverty, and its adverse impact on countries' macroeconomic development. A new global goal for reducing chronic disease death rates over the next 10 years is also introduced.

key messages

» **Chronic disease risks and deaths are increasing rapidly, especially in low and middle income countries**

» **This growing threat is an underappreciated cause of poverty and hinders the macroeconomic development of many countries**

face to face
WITH **CHRONIC DISEASE**

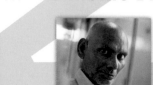

46

K. SRIDHAR REDDY
Paying the price of tobacco use.

68

MARIA SALONIKI
Years in search of the right diagnosis.

80

SHAKEELA BEGUM
To buy or not to buy medication?

1 Chronic diseases: causes and health impacts

The disease profile of the world is changing at an astonishingly fast rate, especially in low and middle income countries. Long-held notions about the nature of chronic diseases, their occurrence, the risk factors underlying them and the populations at risk are no longer valid.

The great epidemics of tomorrow are unlikely to resemble those that have previously swept the world, thanks to progress in infectious disease control. The risk of outbreaks – a new influenza pandemic, for example – will require constant vigilance. But it is the looming epidemics of heart disease, stroke, cancer and other chronic diseases that for the foreseeable future will take the greatest toll in deaths and disability.

It is vitally important that the impending chronic disease pandemic is recognized, understood and acted on urgently.

>> **Chronic diseases will take the lives of over 35 million people in 2005, including many young people and those in middle age**

>> **The total number of people dying from chronic diseases is double that of all infectious diseases (including HIV/AIDS, tuberculosis and malaria), maternal and perinatal conditions, and nutritional deficiencies combined**

>> **80% of chronic disease deaths occur in low and middle income countries and half are in women**

>> **Without action to address the causes, deaths from chronic diseases will increase by 17% between 2005 and 2015**

WHAT ARE CHRONIC DISEASES?

The main chronic diseases discussed in this report are: cardiovascular diseases, mainly heart disease and stroke; cancer; chronic respiratory diseases; and diabetes.

There are many other chronic conditions and diseases that contribute significantly to the burden of disease on individuals, families, societies and countries. Examples include mental disorders, vision and hearing impairment, oral diseases, bone and joint disorders, and genetic disorders. Some will be presented as case studies in this publication to highlight the wide variety of chronic diseases that require continuing attention from all sectors of society. Mental and neurological disorders are important chronic conditions that share a unique set of distinguishing features, and which were reviewed recently by the World Health Organization (1).

TERMINOLOGY

Part of the confusion that surrounds chronic diseases is that they appear under different names in different contexts. Sometimes the term "non-communicable diseases" is used to make the distinction from infectious or "communicable" diseases. Yet several chronic diseases have an infectious component to their cause, such as cervical cancer and liver cancer. "Lifestyle-related" diseases is a term sometimes used to emphasize the contribution of behaviour to the development of chronic diseases. In fact, these diseases are heavily influenced by environmental conditions and are not the result of individual choices alone; "lifestyles" are, of course, equally important for communicable diseases.

For this report, the term "chronic diseases" is preferred because it suggests important shared features:

» the chronic disease epidemics take decades to become fully established – they have their origins at young ages;

» given their long duration, there are many opportunities for prevention;

» they require a long-term and systematic approach to treatment;

» health services must integrate the response to these diseases with the response to acute, infectious diseases.

HEART DISEASE

There are many forms of heart disease. Coronary heart disease, also known as coronary artery disease or ischaemic heart disease, is the leading cause of death globally. This is the form of heart disease considered in this report and it will be referred to simply as heart disease. It is caused by disease of the blood vessels (atherosclerosis) of the heart, usually as part of the process which affects blood vessels more generally. Heart disease, although known for centuries, became common in the early decades of the 20th century in high income countries. The epidemics have now spread worldwide.

STROKE

Stroke is a disease of the brain caused by interference to the blood supply. Stroke and heart disease are the main cardiovascular diseases. There are several types of strokes and the acute events are usually caused by the same long-term disease processes that lead to heart disease; a small proportion of acute events are caused by a blood vessel bursting. Stroke is the main cardiovascular disease in many east Asian countries.

CANCER

Cancer describes a range of diseases in which abnormal cells proliferate and spread out of control. Other terms used are tumours and neoplasms. There are many types of cancer and all organs of the body can become cancerous. Tobacco is the main preventable cause of cancer. The causes of many other cancers are also known, including cervical cancer, skin cancer and oral cancer.

CHRONIC RESPIRATORY DISEASES

Diseases of the lung take many forms. This report focuses on chronic obstructive pulmonary disease and asthma. Chronic obstructive pulmonary disease is caused by airflow limitation that is not fully reversible; asthma is caused by reversible obstruction of the airways.

DIABETES

Diabetes is characterized by raised blood glucose (sugar) levels. This results from a lack of the hormone insulin, which controls blood glucose levels, and/or an inability of the body's tissues to respond properly to insulin (a state called insulin resistance). The most common type of diabetes is type 2, which accounts for about 90% of all diabetes and is largely the result of excessive weight and physical inactivity. Until recently, this type of diabetes was seen only in adults but is now occurring in obese children. The usual childhood form of diabetes (type 1 diabetes) is caused by an absolute lack of insulin and not by obesity. Without insulin, type 1 diabetes is rapidly fatal.

CHRONIC DISEASE PROFILES

This section summarizes the impact of chronic diseases in different populations around the world. Detailed projections for 2005 are presented for males and females of all ages. The data presented are estimated by WHO using standard methods to maximize cross-country comparability; they are not necessarily the official statistics of Member States. For more information on methods of projections for deaths and burden of disease, see Annex 1.

Chronic diseases are projected to take the lives of 35 million people in 2005, which is double the estimate for all infectious diseases combined. Of these chronic disease deaths, 16 million will occur in people under 70 years of age, and 80% will occur in low and middle income countries. Approximately half of the chronic disease deaths occur in females.

THE GLOBAL SITUATION

DEATHS

Approximately 58 million deaths are expected to occur in 2005. It is projected that 35 million – or 60% – of all deaths will be caused by chronic diseases. To put these numbers into perspective, around 17 million deaths – approximately 30% – will be due to infectious diseases (including HIV/AIDS, tuberculosis and malaria), maternal and perinatal conditions, and nutritional deficiencies combined. An additional 5 million deaths – 9% of the total – are expected to result from violence and injuries.

It is often assumed that chronic disease deaths are restricted to older people, but this is not the case. Approximately 16 million chronic disease deaths occur each year in people under 70 years of age. Moreover, chronic disease deaths occur at much earlier ages in low and middle income countries than in high income countries.

The figure on the next page shows the main causes of death worldwide for all ages. Cardiovascular diseases (mainly heart disease and stroke) are the leading cause of death, responsible for 30% of all deaths.

Cancer and chronic respiratory diseases are the other leading causes of chronic disease deaths. The contribution of diabetes is underestimated because although people may live for years with diabetes, their deaths are usually recorded as being caused by heart disease or kidney failure.

Projected main causes of death, worldwide, all ages, 2005

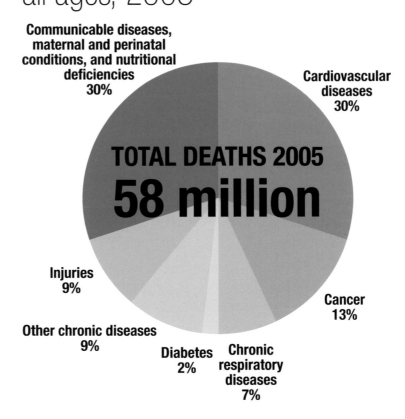

Communicable diseases, maternal and perinatal conditions, and nutritional deficiencies
30%

Cardiovascular diseases
30%

TOTAL DEATHS 2005
58 million

Injuries
9%

Cancer
13%

Other chronic diseases
9%

Diabetes
2%

Chronic respiratory diseases
7%

The number and rates of projected chronic disease deaths in males and females for four age groups are shown in the table on the facing page. The number of deaths is similar in males and females. The death rates for all chronic diseases rise with increasing age but almost 45% of chronic disease deaths occur prematurely, under the age of 70 years.

Projected chronic disease deaths,* worldwide, numbers and rates by age and sex, 2005

Age group	Number of deaths (millions)			Death rates per 100 000		
	Males	Females	Total	Males	Females	Total
0–29	0.8	0.8	1.6	48	47	48
30–59	4	3	7	372	251	311
60–69	4	3	7	2328	1533	1911
70 and over	9	11	20	6981	6102	6467
Total all ages	18	17	35	556	543	549

* Shown to rounded numbers. Components may not add to total exactly owing to rounding.

BURDEN OF DISEASE

As well as a high death toll, chronic diseases also cause disability, often for decades of a person's life. The most widely used summary measure of the burden of disease is the disability adjusted life year (or DALY), which combines the number of years of healthy life lost to premature death with time spent in less than full health. One DALY can be thought of as one lost healthy year of life.

The projected global burden of disease for all ages, as measured by DALYs, is shown in the figure on the right, along with the burden of the leading chronic diseases. Approximately half of the burden of disease will be caused by chronic diseases, 13% by injuries and 39% by communicable diseases, maternal and perinatal conditions, and nutritional deficiencies combined. Cardiovascular diseases are the leading contributor, among the chronic diseases, to the global burden of disease.

The estimated burden of chronic diseases in men and women and for the four age groups is shown in the table on the next page.

Projected main causes of global burden of disease (DALYs), worldwide, all ages, 2005

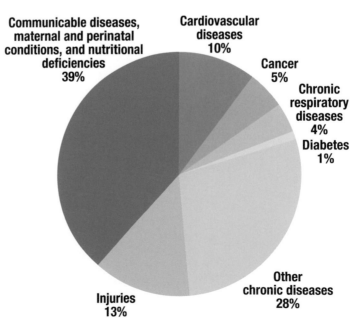

Communicable diseases, maternal and perinatal conditions, and nutritional deficiencies 39%

Cardiovascular diseases 10%

Cancer 5%

Chronic respiratory diseases 4%

Diabetes 1%

Other chronic diseases 28%

Injuries 13%

The number of DALYs caused by chronic disease is greatest in adults aged 30–59 years, and the rates increase with age. Overall, the burden of disease rates are similar in men and women. Approximately 86% of the burden of chronic disease occurs in people under the age of 70 years.

Projected global chronic disease burden (DALYs),* worldwide, numbers and rates by age and sex, 2005

Age group	DALYs (millions)			DALYs per 100 000		
	Males	Females	Total	Males	Females	Total
0–29	112	108	220	6 263	6 380	6 320
30–59	163	143	305	14 088	12 508	13 304
60–69	53	48	101	30 718	25 451	27 965
70 and over	44	55	99	34 570	30 953	32 457
Total all ages	372	354	725	11 470	11 053	11 263

* Shown to rounded numbers. Components may not add to total exactly owing to rounding.

VISUAL IMPAIRMENT

Visual impairment and blindness are examples of chronic conditions whose impact is not captured by death data. In 2002, more than 161 million people were visually impaired, of whom 124 million people had low vision and 37 million were blind as a result of eye diseases. More than 80% of all blindness is in people 50 years of age or older, and women have a significantly higher risk than men.

The highest prevalence of blindness is in the African Region where it reaches 9% among people aged 50 years and older. The lowest prevalence of blindness occurs in the highest income countries of the Americas, South-East Asia and Europe, where it is between 0.4% and 0.6% of people aged 50 years and older.

THE REGIONAL SITUATION

DEATHS

Chronic disease is the leading cause of death in males and females in all WHO regions except Africa, as shown in the figure below.[1]

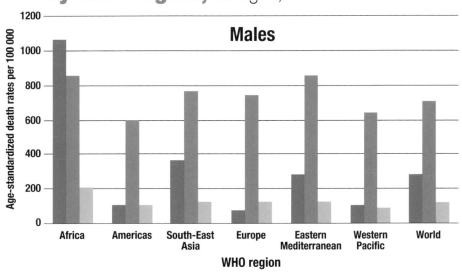

Projected main causes of death by WHO region, all ages, 2005

Males

Age-standardized death rates per 100 000

Africa | Americas | South-East Asia | Europe | Eastern Mediterranean | Western Pacific | World

WHO region

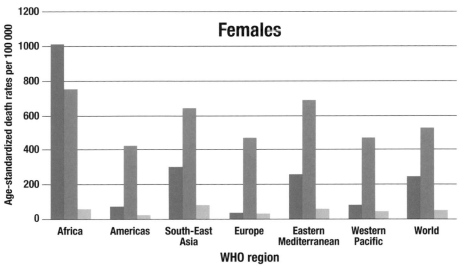

Females

Age-standardized death rates per 100 000

Africa | Americas | South-East Asia | Europe | Eastern Mediterranean | Western Pacific | World

WHO region

■ Communicable diseases, maternal and perinatal conditions, and nutritional deficiencies
■ Chronic diseases
■ Injuries

[1] For a full list of countries by WHO region, see Annex 2.

BURDEN

Chronic diseases are the leading cause of the burden of disease in all regions except Africa; HIV/AIDS is a major contributor in Africa (see figure below).

Projected main causes of the burden of disease (DALYs) by WHO region, all ages, 2005

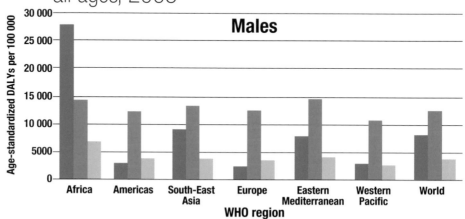

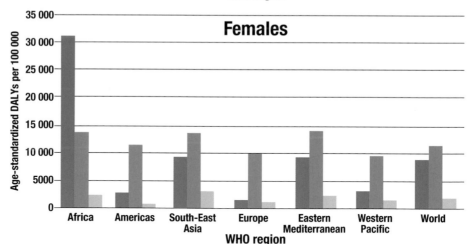

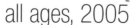
Communicable diseases, maternal and perinatal conditions, and nutritional deficiencies

Chronic diseases

Injuries

THE PATTERN BY COUNTRY INCOME GROUPING

The World Bank categorizes countries into four broad income groupings, based on each country's gross national income (GNI) per capita: low income, middle income (subdivided into lower middle and upper middle) or high income. A full listing of countries is given in Annex 3.

DEATHS

For chronic diseases, the impact is clear: 80% of all chronic disease deaths occur in low and middle income countries, where most of the world's population lives, and the rates are higher than in high income countries. Deaths from chronic diseases occur at earlier ages in low and middle income countries than in high income countries. The figure on the right shows that the age-standardized death rates for chronic diseases are higher in low and middle income countries than in high income countries.

Projected main causes of death by World Bank income group, all ages, 2005

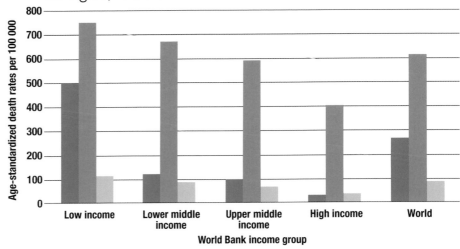

■ Communicable diseases, maternal and perinatal conditions, and nutritional deficiencies
■ Chronic diseases
■ Injuries

BURDEN

Chronic diseases contribute considerably to the disease burden in all income groups. The age-standardized rates are lowest in high income countries.

Projected main causes of burden of disease (DALYs) by World Bank income group, all ages, 2005

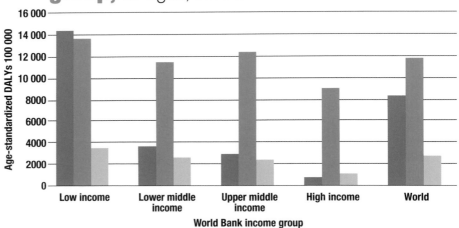

■ Communicable diseases, maternal and perinatal conditions, and nutritional deficiencies
■ Chronic diseases
■ Injuries

COUNTRY PROFILES

DEATHS

The main projected causes of death in 2005 are shown for the nine selected countries in the figure below. Chronic disease death rates are higher than those from communicable diseases, maternal and perinatal conditions, and nutritional deficiencies combined, in all countries except the United Republic of Tanzania and, to a lesser extent, Nigeria.

Remarkably, in low and middle income countries the high death rates in middle-aged people are much higher than those in high income countries (see figure below). This situation is very different from that in Canada and the United Kingdom, where chronic disease deaths now predominantly occur among people in the oldest age group. The death rates in middle-aged people in the Russian Federation are four times those in Canada.

Projected main causes of death
in selected countries, all ages, 2005

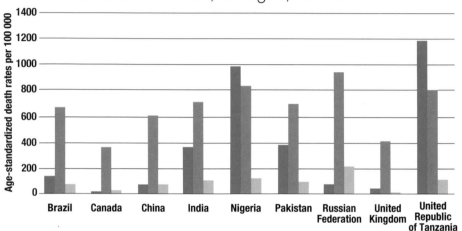

■ Communicable diseases, maternal and perinatal conditions, and nutritional deficiencies
■ Chronic diseases
■ Injuries

Projected chronic disease death rates by country, among people aged 30–69 years, 2005

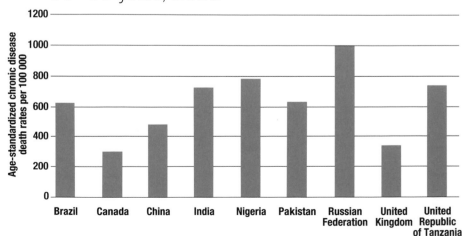

BURDEN

Chronic diseases are the leading cause of the burden of disease in all countries except Nigeria and the United Republic of Tanzania.

Projected main causes of burden of disease (DALYs) in selected countries, all ages, 2005

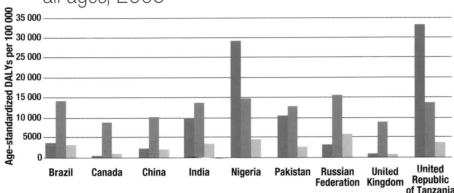

Communicable diseases, maternal and perinatal conditions, and nutritional deficiencies
Chronic diseases
Injuries

SUMMARY

Chronic diseases are the leading cause of death and disease burden worldwide, in all WHO regions except Africa, and in all of the selected countries except Nigeria and the United Republic of Tanzania. Chronic diseases are the leading cause of death in all World Bank income groups. The death and burden of disease rates are similar in men and women and increase with age. Among the selected countries, chronic disease death rates are higher in low and middle income countries than in high income countries. Some 45% of chronic disease deaths and 86% of the burden of chronic diseases occur in people under 70 years of age.

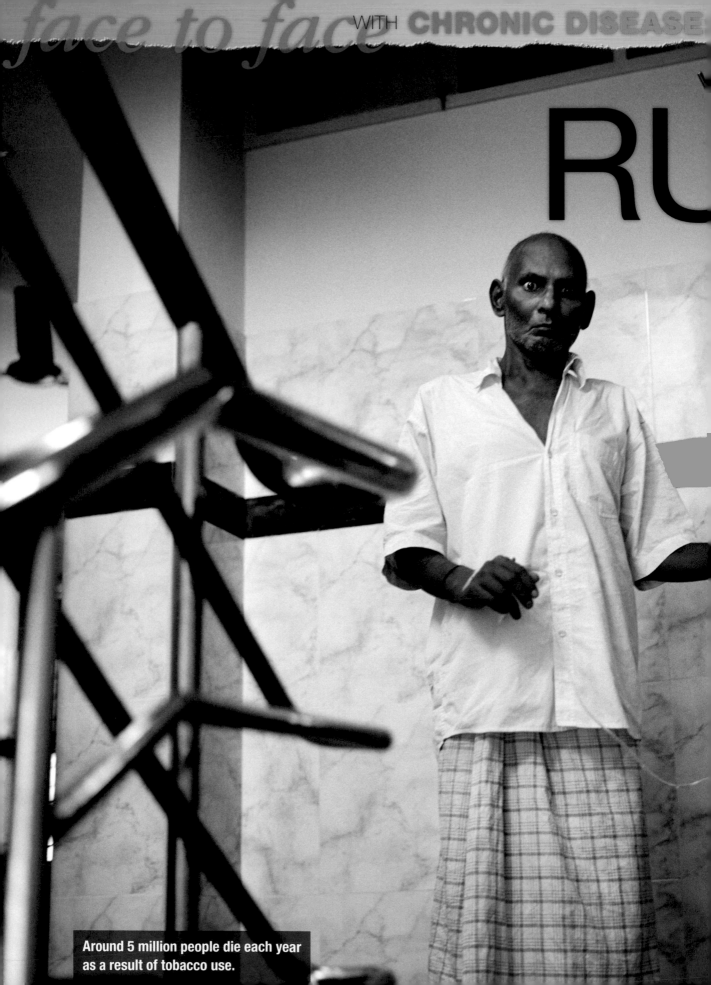

RU

Around 5 million people die each year as a result of tobacco use.

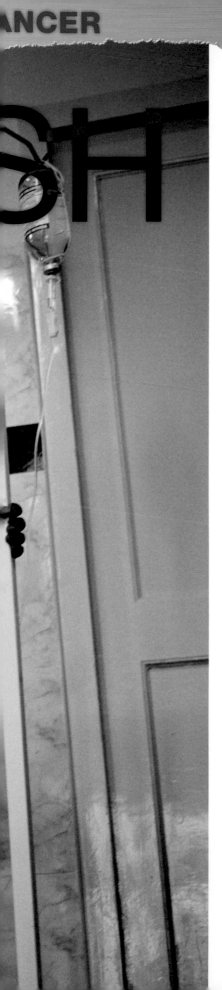

SH HOUR

K. SRIDHAR REDDY

K. SRIDHAR REDDY was on the telephone to his wife when the photographer entered his hospital room. "I'm sorry, it's rush hour, I'll be with you in a minute," he excused himself. Sridhar's wife runs their restaurant while he's undergoing chemotherapy treatment at the Chennai Cancer Institute. "It's my lifeline," the 52-year-old says, looking at his mobile phone.

Name	K. Sridhar Reddy
Age	52
Country	India
Diagnosis	Cancer

Sridhar had a first malignant tumour removed from his right cheek last year and a second one from his throat earlier this year. It's his third hospitalization so far. "Renowned oncologists work here, I'm paying a high price, but I know I'm in good hands," he says, before having a severe coughing fit.

Actually, his doctor doesn't sound as optimistic. Cancer has spread to Sridhar's lungs and liver. "His tobacco use and drinking habits are to blame," the oncologist says, and gives him a year to live at best. Sridhar has been chewing tobacco since his teenage years and drinking alcohol every day for more than 20 years. "Too much stress," Sridhar explains.

Below the surface, Sridhar knows that the future doesn't look bright. He has been borrowing money to pay for his medical bills and now worries that he will never be able to repay the loans.

Sadly, Sridhar died only a short time after he was interviewed.

THE CAUSES OF CHRONIC DISEASES

This section summarizes the extensive evidence on the causes of the chronic disease epidemics. The evidence comes from a full range of studies – laboratory, clinical and population-based – conducted in all regions of the world. The causes (risk factors) of chronic diseases are known; a small set of common risk factors are responsible for most of the main chronic diseases and these risk factors are the same in men and women and in all regions.

THE COMMON CAUSES OF THE MAIN CHRONIC DISEASES

COMMON MODIFIABLE RISK FACTORS

The causes of the main chronic disease epidemics are well established and well known. The most important modifiable risk factors are:

» unhealthy diet and excessive energy intake;

» physical inactivity;

» tobacco use.

These causes are expressed through the intermediate risk factors of raised blood pressure, raised glucose levels, abnormal blood lipids (particularly low density lipoprotein – LDL cholesterol), and overweight (body mass index ≥ 25 kg/m^2) and obesity (body mass index ≥ 30 kg/m^2).

The major modifiable risk factors, in conjunction with the non-modifiable risk factors of age and heredity, explain the majority of new events of heart disease, stroke, chronic respiratory diseases and some important cancers. The relationship between the major modifiable risk factors and the main chronic diseases is similar in all regions of the world.

Causes of chronic diseases

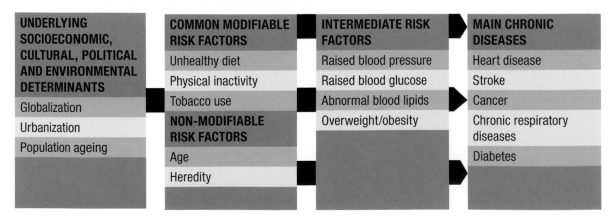

UNDERLYING SOCIOECONOMIC, CULTURAL, POLITICAL AND ENVIRONMENTAL DETERMINANTS	COMMON MODIFIABLE RISK FACTORS	INTERMEDIATE RISK FACTORS	MAIN CHRONIC DISEASES
Globalization	Unhealthy diet	Raised blood pressure	Heart disease
Urbanization	Physical inactivity	Raised blood glucose	Stroke
Population ageing	Tobacco use	Abnormal blood lipids	Cancer
	NON-MODIFIABLE RISK FACTORS	Overweight/obesity	Chronic respiratory diseases
	Age		Diabetes
	Heredity		

OTHER RISK FACTORS

Many more risk factors for chronic diseases have been identified, but they account for a smaller proportion of chronic disease.

Harmful alcohol use is an important contributor to the global burden of disease. It has been estimated to result in 3% of global deaths and 4% of the global burden of disease, almost half of which being the result of unintentional and intentional injuries. The relationship of alcohol use to chronic disease is complex. The health consequences of excessive alcohol use include liver cirrhosis (damage to liver cells); pancreatitis (inflammation of the pancreas); and various cancers, including cancer of the liver, mouth, throat, larynx and esophagus. On the other hand, current evidence from epidemiological and experimental studies suggests that a very low consumption of alcohol has a protective effect against the development of cardiovascular diseases. This protective effect only becomes important as the risk of cardiovascular disease increases in middle-aged and older people. At younger ages the adverse effects of alcohol use, especially violence and injuries, outweigh the benefits.

Other risk factors for chronic disease include infectious agents that are responsible for cervical and liver cancers, and some environmental factors such as air pollution, which contribute to a range of chronic diseases including asthma and other chronic respiratory diseases. Psychosocial and genetic factors also play a role.

CHILDHOOD RISK: A WORRYING TREND

There is now extensive evidence from many countries that conditions before birth and in early childhood influence health in adult life. For example, low birth weight is now known to be associated with increased rates of high blood pressure, heart disease, stroke and diabetes (2).

Children cannot choose the environment in which they live, including their diet, living situation, and exposure to tobacco smoke. They also have a very limited ability to understand the long-term consequences of their behaviour. Yet it is precisely during this crucial phase that many health behaviours are shaped. Young tobacco smokers, for example, may acquire the habit and become dependent well before reaching adulthood.

Rates of tobacco use among 13–15 year-olds are higher than previously expected. According to the Global Youth Tobacco Survey and Global School-based Student Health Survey, current tobacco use among males in this age group is 29% in India, 21% in Brazil, and 14% in China. Many children begin smoking before the age of 10 years.

Childhood obesity is associated with a higher chance of premature death and disability in adulthood. Worryingly, approximately 22 million children under the age of five years are obese. While affecting every country, overweight and obesity in children are particularly common in North America, the United Kingdom, and south-western Europe. In Malta and the United States, over a quarter of children aged 10–16 years are overweight. In the United Kingdom, the prevalence of overweight in children aged 2 to 10 years rose from 23% to 28% between 1995 and 2003.

Obesity is a known risk factor for type 2 diabetes. Until recently type 2 diabetes was mainly a disease of adults. The first cases of type 2 diabetes in young people were recognized in the United States in the 1970s. Fifteen years ago, they accounted for less than 3% of all cases of new-onset diabetes in children and adolescents, whereas today they account for up to 45% of new-onset cases. Subsequent studies conducted in Asia and Europe have revealed a similar pattern, and, more recently, reports on type 2 diabetes in children and adolescents have begun to mount worldwide (3).

A life course approach to chronic diseases

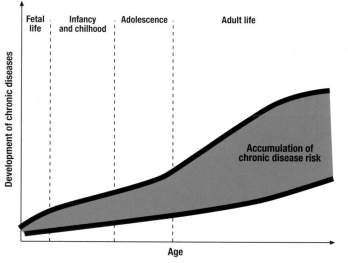

RISK ACCUMULATION

Ageing is an important marker of the accumulation of modifiable risks for chronic disease: the impact of risk factors increases over the life course. A key lesson from many wealthy countries is that it is possible to delay deaths from chronic diseases by several decades, thereby avoiding deaths among middle-aged people. Successful interventions in middle and older age will reap major short-term benefits. In the longer term, interventions early in life have the potential to reduce substantially the chronic disease pandemic.

UNDERLYING DETERMINANTS

The underlying determinants of chronic diseases – the "causes of the causes" – are a reflection of the major forces driving social, economic and cultural change – globalization, urbanization, population ageing, and the general policy environment. The role of poverty is described in the next chapter.

Globalization refers to the increasing interconnectedness of countries and the openness of borders to ideas, people, commerce and financial capital. Globalization drives chronic disease population risks in complex ways, both directly and indirectly. The health-related advantages of globalization include the introduction of modern technologies, such as information and communication technologies for health-care systems.

The negative health-related effects of globalization include the trend known as the "nutrition transition": populations in low and middle income countries are now consuming diets high in total energy, fats, salt and sugar. The increased consumption of these foods in these countries is driven partly by shifts in demand-side factors, such as increased income and reduced time to prepare food. Supply-side determinants include increased production, promotion and marketing of processed foods and those high in fat, salt and sugar, as well as tobacco and other products with adverse effects on population health status. A significant proportion of global marketing is now targeted at children and underlies unhealthy behaviour.

The widespread belief that chronic diseases are only "diseases of affluence" is incorrect. Chronic disease risks become widespread much earlier in a country's economic development than is usually realized. For example, population levels of body mass index and total cholesterol increase rapidly as poor countries become richer and national income rises. They remain steady once a certain level of national income is reached, before eventually declining (see next chapter) (4).

In the second half of the 20th century, the proportion of people in Africa, Asia and Latin America living in urban areas rose from 16% to 50%. Urbanization creates conditions in which people are exposed to new products, technologies, and marketing of unhealthy goods, and in which they adopt less physically active types of employment. Unplanned urban sprawl can further reduce physical activity levels by discouraging walking or bicycling.

As well as globalization and urbanization, rapid population ageing is occurring worldwide. The total number of people aged 70 years or more worldwide is expected to increase from 269 million in 2000 to 1 billion in 2050. High income countries will see their elderly population (defined as people 70 years of age and older) increase from 93 million to 217 million over this period, while in low and middle income countries the increase will be 174 million to 813 million – more than 466%.

The general policy environment is another crucial determinant of population health. Policies by central and local government on food, agriculture, trade, media advertising, transport, urban design and the built environment shape opportunities for people to make healthy choices. In an unsupportive policy environment it is difficult for people, especially those in deprived populations, to benefit from existing knowledge on the causes and prevention of the main chronic diseases.

THE HEALTH IMPACT OF THE MAIN RISK FACTORS

The contribution of risk factors to death and disease is estimated by calculating the current "attributable" mortality and burden of disease (DALYs) caused by past exposure to the main risk factors over and above the minimum possible risk factor exposure.

Chronic disease risk factors are a leading cause of the death and disease burden in all countries, regardless of their economic development status. The leading risk factor globally is raised blood pressure, followed by tobacco use, raised total cholesterol, and low fruit and vegetable consumption. The major risk factors together account for around 80% of deaths from heart disease and stroke (5).

Each year at least:

» 4.9 million people die as a result of tobacco use;

» 1.9 million people die as a result of physical inactivity;

» 2.7 million people die as a result of low fruit and vegetable consumption;

» 2.6 million people die as a result of being overweight or obese;

» 7.1 million people die as a result of raised blood pressure;

» 4.4 million people die as a result of raised total cholesterol levels (5).

Further analyses using 2002 death estimates show that among the nine selected countries, the proportion of deaths from all causes of disease attributable to raised systolic blood pressure (greater than 115 mm Hg) is highest in the Russian Federation with similar patterns in men and women, representing more than 5 million years of life lost. A similar picture emerges when the contribution of the risk factors to the burden of disease (DALYs) is estimated.

Percent attributable deaths from raised blood pressure by country, all ages, 2002

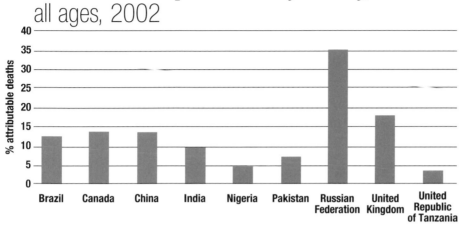

The proportion of deaths attributed to raised body mass index (greater than 21 kg/m^2) for all causes is highest in the Russian Federation, accounting for over 14% of total deaths, followed by Canada, the United Kingdom, and Brazil, where it accounts for 8–10% of total deaths. The pattern is similar for men and women and for the attributable burden of disease (DALYs).

Percent of attributable deaths from raised body mass index by country, all ages, 2002

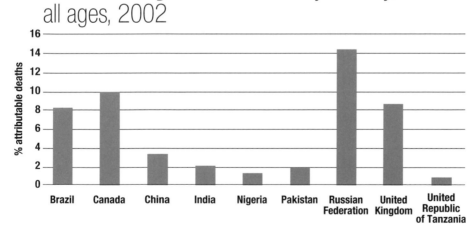

The estimates of mortality and burden of disease attributed to the main modifiable risk factors, as illustrated above, show that in all nine countries raised blood pressure and raised body mass index are of great public health significance, most of all in the Russian Federation.

RISK FACTOR PROJECTIONS CASE STUDY: OVERWEIGHT AND OBESITY

This section describes the patterns of overweight and obesity projected for 2005 to 2015 globally, regionally, and in the selected countries. The data come from the WHO Global InfoBase (*6*) which collects, stores, and disseminates data on the major chronic disease risk factors, and uses methods developed for the Comparative Risk Assessment Study (*5, 7*). Projections for other risk factors are available on the WHO Global InfoBase.

GLOBAL PROFILE

Globally, in 2005, it is estimated that over 1 billion people are overweight, including 805 million women, and that over 300 million people are obese. Maps of the worldwide prevalence of overweight in adult women for 2005 and 2015 are shown opposite. If current trends continue, average levels of body mass index are projected to increase in almost all countries. By 2015, it is estimated that over 1.5 billion people will be overweight.

Projected prevalence of overweight (BMI*≥25 kg/m²), women aged 30 and above, 2005

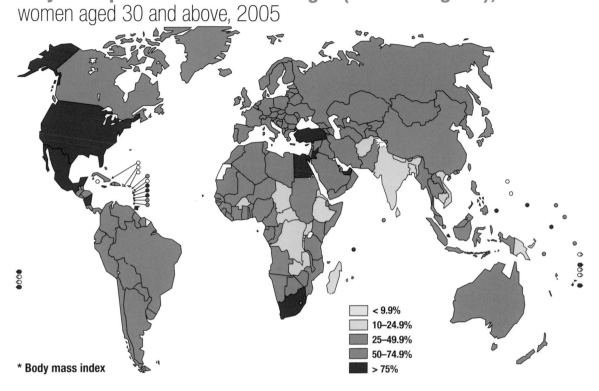

* Body mass index

	< 9.9%
	10–24.9%
	25–49.9%
	50–74.9%
	> 75%

Projected prevalence of overweight (BMI*≥25 kg/m²), women aged 30 and above, 2015

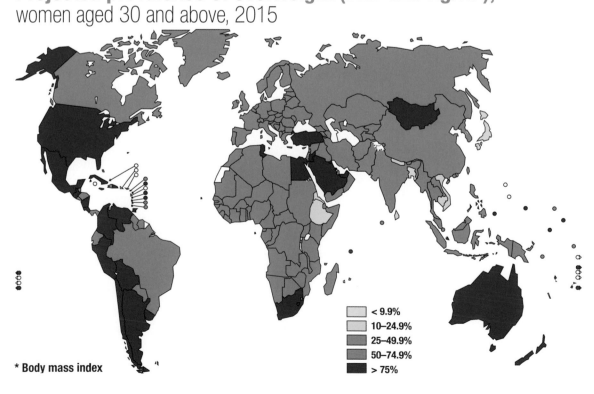

* Body mass index

	< 9.9%
	10–24.9%
	25–49.9%
	50–74.9%
	> 75%

PROJECTIONS BY COUNTRY INCOME GROUP

BODY MASS INDEX

Projected prevalence of overweight (BMI*≥25 kg/m²), women aged 30 years or more, by World Bank income group, 2005–2015

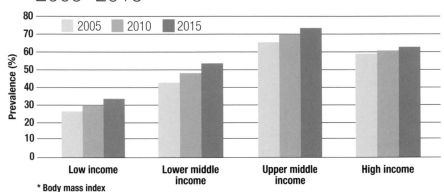

* Body mass index

In both men and women, there is expected to be a steady increase in average body mass index, and associated overweight and obesity levels will rise regardless of income grouping. The largest increase is projected to be in women from upper middle income countries. This group has already overtaken women in high income countries.

Projected prevalence of overweight (BMI*≥25 kg/m²), women aged 30 years or more, selected countries, 2005–2015

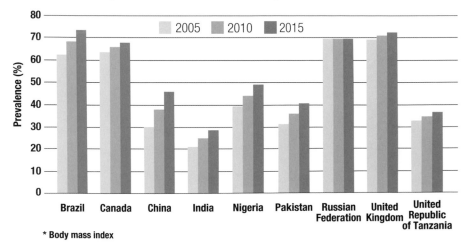

* Body mass index

COUNTRY PROFILES

Once associated only with high income countries, overweight and obesity are now also prevalent in low and middle income countries. A rapid increase in overweight is expected in all of the selected countries except the United Republic of Tanzania, although clear differences remain between countries and between men and women. The highest projected prevalence of overweight in women in the selected countries in 2015 will be in Brazil, followed by the United Kingdom, the Russian Federation and Canada. The most rapid increase, albeit from a low level, is expected in Chinese women.

PROJECTIONS OF FUTURE DEATHS

In this section, death projections for 2015 are presented for the world population, by country income group and for the nine selected countries. The projections are based on current country-level comparable estimates for 2002, and take into account expected changes in death rates associated with continued economic development, projected trends in HIV/AIDS and population ageing. For more information, see Annex 1.

In general, deaths from chronic diseases are projected to increase between 2005 and 2015, while at the same time deaths from communicable diseases, maternal and perinatal conditions, and nutritional deficiencies combined are projected to decrease. The projected increase in the burden of chronic diseases worldwide is largely driven by population ageing, supplemented by the large numbers of people who are now exposed to chronic disease risk factors.

There will be a total of 64 million deaths in 2015:

» 17 million people will die from communicable diseases, maternal and perinatal conditions, and nutritional deficiencies combined;

» 41 million people will die from chronic diseases;

» Cardiovascular diseases will remain the single leading cause of death, with an estimated 20 million people dying, mainly from heart disease and stroke;

» Deaths from chronic diseases will increase by 17% between 2005 and 2015, from 35 million to 41 million.

SELECTED COUNTRIES

Overall, death rates in the nine selected countries are projected to decrease for communicable diseases, maternal and perinatal conditions and nutritional deficiencies. The exception is HIV/AIDS, for which substantial increases are projected to occur between 2005 and 2015 in all countries except Canada and the United Kingdom.

In all countries except Nigeria and the United Republic of Tanzania, chronic diseases will be the leading cause of death in 2015.

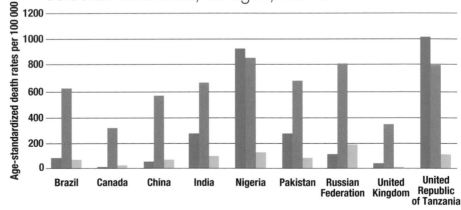

Projected main causes of death, selected countries, all ages, 2015

Age-standardized death rates per 100 000

Brazil, Canada, China, India, Nigeria, Pakistan, Russian Federation, United Kingdom, United Republic of Tanzania

■ Communicable diseases, maternal and perinatal conditions, and nutritional deficiencies
■ Chronic diseases
▪ Injuries

A VISION FOR THE FUTURE: REDUCING DEATHS AND IMPROVING LIVES

Recent progress in public health has helped people in many parts of the world to live longer and healthier lives. There is abundant evidence of how the use of existing knowledge has led to major improvements in the life expectancy and quality of life of middle-aged and older people. Yet as this chapter has shown, approximately four out of five chronic disease deaths now occur in low and middle income countries. People in these countries are also more prone to dying prematurely than those in high income countries.

The results presented in this chapter suggest that a global goal for preventing chronic disease is needed to generate the sustained actions required to reduce the disease burden. The target for this proposed goal is an additional 2% reduction in chronic disease death rates annually over the next 10 years to 2015. The indicators for the measurement of success towards this goal are the number of chronic disease deaths averted and the number of healthy life years gained.

This target was developed based on the achievements of several countries, such as Poland, which achieved a 6–10% annual reduction in cardiovascular deaths during the 1990s (8). Similar results have been realized over the past three decades in a number of countries in which comprehensive programmes have been introduced, such as Australia, Canada, New Zealand, the United Kingdom, and the United States (9–11).

This global goal aims to reduce death rates in addition to the declines already projected for many chronic diseases – and would result in 36 million chronic disease deaths averted by 2015. This represents an increase of approximately 500 million life years gained for the world over the 10-year period. Cardiovascular diseases and cancers are the diseases for which most deaths would be averted. Most of the deaths averted from specific chronic diseases would be in low and middle income countries as demonstrated by the top figure, opposite (12).

Projected cumulative deaths averted by achieving the global goal, by World Bank income group, 2006–2015

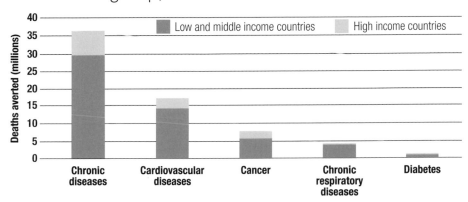

Every death averted is a bonus, but the goal contains an additional positive feature: almost half of these averted deaths would be in men and women under 70 years of age (see figure below). Extending their lives for the benefit of the individuals concerned, their families and communities is in itself the worthiest of goals. It also supports the overall goal of chronic disease prevention and control, which is to delay mortality from these diseases and to promote healthy ageing of people everywhere.

Chronic disease deaths, projected from 2005 to 2015 and with global goal scenario, for people aged 70 years or less

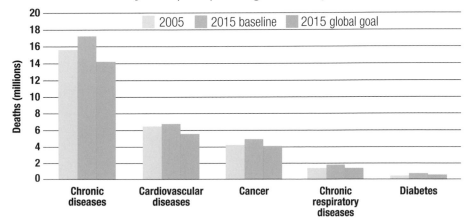

This goal is ambitious and adventurous, but it is neither extravagant nor unrealistic. The means to achieve it, based on the evidence and best practices from countries that have already made such improvements, such as the United Kingdom and the other countries referred to above, are outlined in Parts Three and Four of this report.

CONCLUSION

Confusion and long-held misunderstandings about the nature of chronic diseases, their prevalence, the populations at risk, and the risk factors themselves are barriers to progress and prevention. What might have been true – or thought to be true – 30, 20 or even 10 years ago is no longer the case.

The health of the world is generally improving, with fewer people dying from infectious diseases and therefore in many cases living long enough to develop chronic diseases. Increases in the causes of chronic diseases, including unhealthy diet, physical inactivity and tobacco use are leading to people developing chronic diseases at younger ages in the increasingly urban environments of low and middle income countries. Disturbing evidence of this impact in many of these countries is steadily growing. They are ill equipped to handle the demands for care and treatment that chronic diseases place on their health systems and so people die at younger ages than in high income countries.

Individuals and their families in all countries struggle to cope with the impact of chronic diseases, and it is the poorest who are the most vulnerable. The links between chronic diseases and poverty are examined in the next chapter.

Chronic diseases and poverty

2

The chronic disease burden is concentrated among the poor

Poor people are more vulnerable for several reasons, including increased exposure to risks and decreased access to health services

Chronic diseases can cause poverty in individuals and families, and draw them into a downward spiral of worsening disease and poverty

Investment in chronic disease prevention programmes is essential for many low and middle income countries struggling to reduce poverty

Chronic diseases and poverty are interconnected in a vicious cycle. This chapter explains how, in almost all countries, it is the poorest people who are most at risk of developing chronic diseases and dying prematurely from them. Poor people are more vulnerable for several reasons, including greater exposure to risks and decreased access to health services.

Poverty and worsening of already existing poverty are also caused by chronic diseases. Once again, it is people and families who are already poor who are most likely to suffer, because chronic diseases are likely to ruin a family's economic prospects. Poverty can be divided into *extreme* (when households cannot meet basic needs for survival), *moderate* (in which basic needs are barely met), and *relative* poverty (in which household income is less than a proportion of average national income). All of these poverty types adversely affect health. Poverty is found in every country, but unlike moderate and relative poverty, extreme poverty occurs mainly in low income countries (*13*).

Wealth enables people to avoid most of the risks of developing chronic disease, and to obtain access to health care. However, even within high income countries, psychosocial factors, for example lack of social support and perceived lack of control, are strongly related to the risk of chronic diseases (*14*). At the same time, in some countries, evidence clearly links growing national income with increases in obesity and high cholesterol levels across the population. Alarmingly, the evidence also reveals that this trend occurs at an earlier stage of socioeconomic development than has been previously assumed. As countries develop economically, some risk factors appear to affect wealthier populations first, although they quickly concentrate among the poor.

FROM POVERTY TO CHRONIC DISEASES

Poverty and social exclusion increase the risks of developing a chronic disease, developing complications and dying. The resulting health inequalities have been widening over the past two decades. In some countries at an early stage of economic development, wealthy members of society report more chronic disease than poorer members – it is unclear, however, whether this is because they develop more chronic diseases, or because they survive with them longer owing to their ability to access health services. In all countries, poor people are more likely to die after developing a chronic disease. In most countries, health inequalities have been widening over recent decades (*15, 16*).

WHY THE POOR ARE MORE VULNERABLE

The poor are more vulnerable to chronic diseases because of material deprivation and psychosocial stress, higher levels of risk behaviour, unhealthy living conditions and limited access to good-quality health care (see sidebar figure on the next page). Once disease is established, poor people are more likely to suffer adverse consequences than wealthier people. This is especially true of women, as they are often more vulnerable to the effects of social inequality and poverty, and less able to access resources.

WIDENING GAPS IN HIGH INCOME COUNTRIES

The gap between rich and poor has been widening in many wealthy countries in recent years. In Denmark, England and Wales, Finland, Italy, Norway, and Sweden inequalities in mortality increased between the 1980s and the 1990s. These widening inequalities have been attributed to two important changes.

The first is that cardiovascular disease death rates declined among wealthy members of these societies, explaining about half of the widening gap. This might have been a result of faster changes in health behaviour in these groups and/or better access to health-care interventions.

Second, widening inequalities in other causes of death (lung cancer, breast cancer, respiratory disease, gastrointestinal disease and injuries) resulted from increasing rates of mortality among poorer groups. Rising rates of lung cancer and deaths from chronic respiratory disease indicate the delayed effects of rising tobacco use among poorer members of society (*16*).

HIGHER LEVELS OF RISK BEHAVIOUR

The immediate cause of inequalities in chronic diseases is the existence of higher levels of risk factors among the poor. The poor and people with less education are more likely to use tobacco products, consume energy-dense and high-fat food, be physically inactive, and be overweight or obese (*17*).

This social and economic difference in risk factor prevalence is particularly striking in high income countries, but is also rapidly becoming a prominent feature of low and middle income countries (*18, 19*).

Poor people and those with less education are more likely to maintain risk behaviour for several reasons. These include inequality of opportunities, such as general education; psychosocial stress; limited choice of consumption patterns; inadequate access to health care and health education; and vulnerability to the adverse effects of globalization.

Aggressive marketing of harmful products, such as tobacco, sustain the demand for these products among those who have fewer opportunities to substitute unhealthy habits with healthier and often more expensive options.

From poverty to chronic diseases

Material deprivation and psychosocial stress

▼

Constrained choices and higher levels of risk behaviour

▼

Increased risk of disease

▼

Disease onset

▼

Reduced access to care

▼

Reduced opportunity to prevent complications

In middle and high income countries, the poor tend to be more obese than the wealthy, which has been viewed as something of a paradox. It is likely that several factors contribute to this relationship, but one explanation is that "energy-dense" foods, such as fried or processed foods, tend to cost less on a per-calorie basis when compared with fresh fruit and vegetables (20).

COMMUNITY DEPRIVATION

Economic deprivation often leads to reduced access to the requirements of a healthy life, including affordable, nutritious foods, adequate housing and health care, and a good social support network such as family, friends and community groups. Many people live in areas that cause them to be concerned for their safety, thereby reducing opportunities for outdoor physical activities. People living in disadvantaged communities marked by sprawling development are likely to walk less and weigh more than others. People from deprived communities suffer more from cardiovascular diseases than residents of more affluent communities, even taking into account other known risk factors (21, 22).

POOR ACCESS TO QUALITY HEALTH CARE AND MEDICATIONS

Inadequate access to good-quality health services, including diagnostic and clinical prevention services, is a significant cause of the social and economic inequalities in the burden of chronic diseases. The poor face several health-care barriers including financial constraints, lack of proximity and/or availability of transport to health-care centres, and poor responsiveness from the health-care system (23, 24).

Financial considerations can act as barriers to health-care access. Some people are unable to afford out-of-pocket charges for health care and might forfeit their wages by missing work. Transport costs can also prevent people from seeking care, especially those who must travel long distances to health centres. The poor usually have much more limited access to prescription drugs (25).

Even when health services are subsidized by the government or provided free in low and middle income countries, it is the wealthier who gain more from such services. Findings from South Africa, for example, showed that among people with high blood pressure, the wealthiest 30% of the population was more than twice as likely to have received treatment as the poorest 40% (26).

SPOTLIGHT
RISK FACTORS IN THE UNITED REPUBLIC OF TANZANIA

The United Republic of Tanzania demonstrates a mixed picture with regard to risk factors. Higher social and economic status is associated with higher body mass index, but lower systolic blood pressure and lower prevalence of tobacco use. This finding supports the idea that as countries develop economically, different risk factors affect different social and economic classes at different rates (19).

In rural areas, health workers and health centres are more dispersed, and health services might be of lower quality than in urban health centres.

The poor and marginalized are often confronted with insufficient responsiveness from the health-care system. Communication barriers may significantly decrease effective access to health services and inhibit the degree to which a patient can benefit from such services. Migrants, for example, often face language and other cultural barriers.

GENDER INEQUALITY

Social inequality, poverty and inequitable access to resources, including health care, result in a high burden of chronic diseases among women worldwide, particularly very poor women.

In general, women tend to live longer with chronic disease than men, though they are often in poor health. The costs associated with health care, including user fees, are a barrier to women's use of services. Women's income is lower than that of men, and they have less control over household resources. They may not be able to pay for treatment unless there is agreement from senior members (whether male or female) of the household. Women's workload in the home and their caregiving roles when other family members are ill are also significant factors in delaying decisions to seek treatment. In areas where women have limited mobility, they may be unable to travel to health centres (27).

SPOTLIGHT
AFFORDABILITY OF MEDICINES IN THE RUSSIAN FEDERATION

In 1994, the main obstacle to obtaining medicines in the Russian Federation was unavailability, for both rural and urban populations. Almost 75% of people who could not obtain medicines reported unavailability as the main reason, and only 20–25% could not afford them. However, since then the situation has changed dramatically: availability of medicines has significantly improved but they have become far less affordable. By 2000, 65–70% of people who could not obtain medicines reported unaffordability as the main reason, while unavailability accounted for only 20% of the access gap (29).

SPOTLIGHT
BLINDNESS IN WOMEN

In low and middle income countries, the leading causes of blindness – cataract and trachomatous trichiasis – occur more frequently in women. Population-based surveys of blindness in Africa, Asia and many high income countries suggest that women account for 65% of all blind people worldwide. At the same time, women do not have equal access to surgery for eye diseases. Cataract blindness could be reduced by about 13% if women received cataract surgery at the same rate as men. Women are more likely to wait until they are blind to undergo surgery. The decision to delay treatment is often influenced by the cost of the surgery, inability to travel to a surgical facility, differences in the perceived value of surgery (cataract is often viewed as an inevitable consequence of ageing and women are less likely to experience support within the family to seek care), and lack of access to health information (28).

FROM CHRONIC DISEASES TO POVERTY

The previous section illustrated that the poor are more likely both to develop chronic diseases and to suffer more from the negative consequences of chronic disease. This section describes how chronic diseases cause poverty and draw individuals and their families into a downward spiral of worsening disease and impoverishment.

THE CYCLE OF POVERTY

An important cause of poverty in low and middle income countries is the death or severe illness of a family's primary income earner. Out of 125 case studies summarized in the World Bank's publication *Voices of the poor crying out for change*, illness, injury or death was the most common trigger of households' impoverishment (*32*). In Bangladesh, for example, of those households that moved into the status "always poor", all reported death or severe disabling diseases as one of the main causes.

Chronic diseases inflict an enormous direct and indirect economic burden on the poor, and push many people and their families into poverty. Existing knowledge underestimates the implications of chronic diseases for poverty and the potential that chronic disease prevention and health promotion have for alleviating poverty in low and middle income countries (*33*).

DIRECT ECONOMIC IMPACT

CATASTROPHIC EXPENDITURE

Direct costs related to chronic disease include out-of-pocket payments for health services and medications. Ongoing health care-related expenses for chronic diseases are a major problem for many poor people. Acute chronic disease-related events – such as a heart attack or stroke – can be disastrously expensive, and are so for millions of people.

People who fall ill often face a dire choice: either to suffer and perhaps die without treatment, or to seek treatment and push their family into poverty. Those who suffer from long-standing chronic diseases are in the worst situation, because the costs of medical care are incurred over a long period of time (*34*).

SPOTLIGHT
BARRIERS TO TREATMENT IN JAMAICA

In Jamaica 59% of people with chronic diseases experienced financial difficulties because of their illness, and a high proportion of people admitting such difficulties avoided some medical treatment as a result (*30*).

SPOTLIGHT
MEDICAL EXPENSES IN INDIA

People in India with diabetes spend a significant portion of their annual income on medical care. The poorest people – those who can least afford the cost – spend the greatest proportion of their income on medical care. On average, they spend 25% of their annual income on private care, compared with 4% in high income groups (*31*).

TOBACCO USE

For various reasons, tobacco use tends to be higher among the poor than wealthier members of society, and they therefore spend relatively more on tobacco products. Spending money on tobacco deprives people of education opportunities that could help lift them out of poverty and also leads to greater health-care costs.

INDIRECT ECONOMIC IMPACT

Chronic diseases have an indirect impact on people's economic status and employment opportunities in the long term. Indirect costs include:

» reduction in income owing to lost productivity from illness or death;

» the cost of adult household members caring for those who are ill;

» reduction in future earnings by the selling of assets to cope with direct costs and unpredictable expenditures;

» lost opportunities for young members of the household who leave school in order to care for adults who are ill or to help the household economy (35).

REDUCTION IN INCOME

In most high income countries, people with chronic diseases and disabilities are protected by social security systems, yet they still experience adverse economic consequences. However, in low and middle income countries disability insurance systems are either underdeveloped or nonexistent.

The illness of a main income earner in low and middle income countries significantly reduces overall household income. People who have chronic diseases are not fully able to compensate for income lost during periods of illness when they are in relatively good health (36).

SALE OF HOUSEHOLD POSSESSIONS

Chronic diseases affect household investment and consumption patterns. Households often sell their possessions to cover lost income and health-care costs. In the short term, this might help poor households to cope with urgent medical costs, but in the long term it has a negative effect: the selling of productive assets – property that produces income – increases the vulnerability of households and drives them into poverty. Such changes in the investment pattern of households are more likely to occur when chronic diseases require long-term, costly treatment (36).

SPOTLIGHT
ECONOMIC IMPACT OF TOBACCO USE

It is estimated that over 10.5 million people in Bangladesh who are malnourished could have an adequate diet if money spent on tobacco were spent on food instead, saving the lives of 350 children under the age of five years each day. The poorest households in Bangladesh spend almost 10 times as much on tobacco as on education (37).

In countries such as Bulgaria, Egypt, Indonesia, Myanmar and Nepal, household expenditure surveys show that low income households spend 5–15% of their disposable income on tobacco (37).

In India, people are more likely to borrow money and sell their assets during hospitalization if they are tobacco users. The same is true if they are nonusers but belong to households that use tobacco (38).

In the United Kingdom, the average cost of monthly health insurance premiums for a 35-year-old female smoker is 65% higher than the cost for a nonsmoker. Male smokers pay 70% higher health insurance premiums than nonsmokers (37).

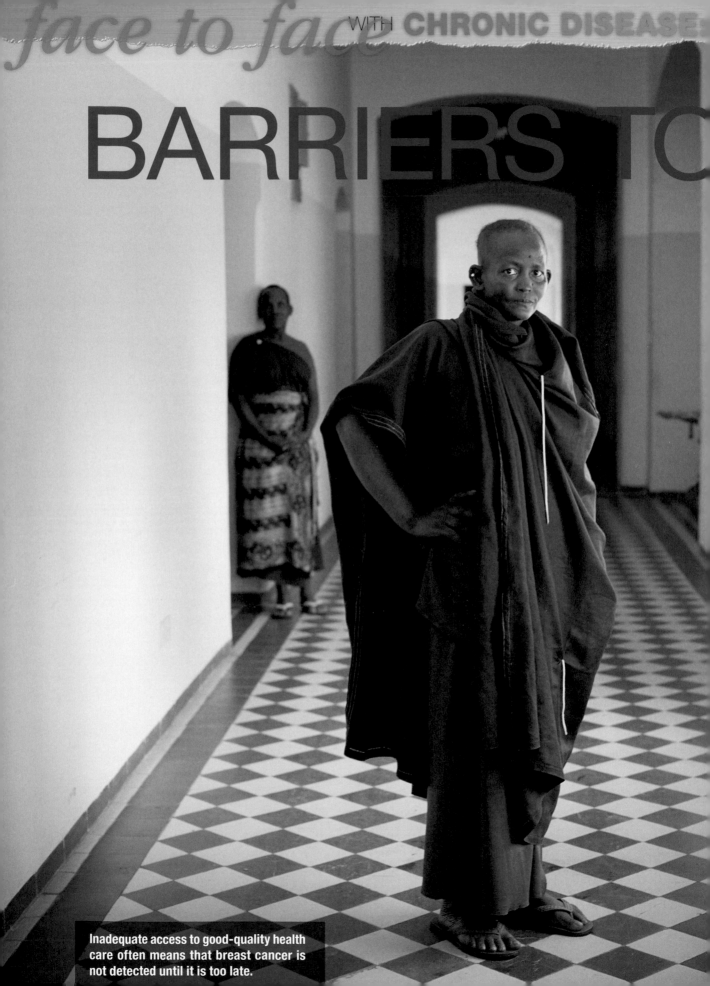

BARRIERS TO

Inadequate access to good-quality health care often means that breast cancer is not detected until it is too late.

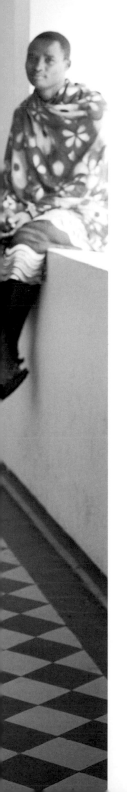

MARIA SALONIKI
HEALTH CARE

MARIA SALONIKI CAN HARDLY REMEMBER how many times she went to the local traditional healer, how many doctors in clinics and dispensaries she consulted between two hospitalizations, how many words she used to describe her pain. But one thing she clearly remembers is that each time she returned home without receiving adequate treatment and care.

Name	Maria Saloniki
Age	60
Country	United Republic of Tanzania
Diagnosis	Breast cancer

Today, this livestock keeper and mother of 10 children is fighting for her life at the Ocean Road Cancer Institute in Dar es Salaam. It took Maria more than three years to discover the words to describe her pain – breast cancer – and to receive the treatment she desperately needs. "It all started with a swollen armpit and a bad fever," she recalls.

In fact, between these first symptoms and chemotherapy treatment, Maria was prescribed herb ointments on several occasions, has been on antibiotics twice and heard from more than one health professional that they couldn't do anything for her. The 60-year-old even travelled to Nairobi, Kenya to seek treatment, but it wasn't until later, in Dar es Salaam, that a biopsy revealed her disease.

Maria's story is sadly common in the understaffed and poorly equipped hospital ward she shares with 30 other cancer patients. Her husband, who now works day and night to pay for her medicine and feed their children, can't afford both the treatment costs and the bus fare to come and visit her. The family has one year to pay back a substantial loan to its tribe.

INTERGENERATIONAL IMPACT

The death or illness of adults from chronic disease can lead to the impoverishment of their children. To compensate for the lost productivity of a sick or disabled adult, children are often removed from school; this deprives them of the opportunity to study and gain qualifications.

The fact that an adult family member has a chronic disease can also have direct health implications for children. According to a study in Bangladesh, for example, the relative risk of a severely malnourished child coming from a household with an incapacitated income earner is 2.5 times greater than that of households which are not in such a situation (40).

CHRONIC DISEASES AND THE MILLENNIUM DEVELOPMENT GOALS

In September 2000, the largest-ever gathering of Heads of State ushered in the new millennium by adopting the UN Millennium Declaration. The Declaration, endorsed by 189 countries, was then translated into a roadmap setting out goals to be reached by 2015. Health is central to the achievement of the Millennium Development Goals (MDGs), and three goals relate specifically to health issues: those concerned with reducing child mortality, improving maternal health, and combating HIV/AIDS, malaria and other diseases.

The MDGs have successfully focused attention on the plight of the world's poorest children and mothers, and on some infectious disease epidemics. However, chronic diseases – the major cause of death in almost all countries – have not been included within the global targets; although as a recent WHO publication on health and the MDGs has recognized, there is scope for doing so within Goal 6 (Combat HIV/AIDS, malaria and other diseases) (41). Health more broadly, including chronic disease prevention, contributes to poverty reduction and hence Goal 1 (Eradicate extreme poverty and hunger).

A recent World Bank study has found that the generic MDG targets are only of limited relevance for countries in eastern Europe and the former Soviet Union. The implications are relevant to many other countries that face a notable chronic disease burden.

In the countries studied, reduction of adult mortality to the level found in the European Union would have the greatest impact on life expectancy at birth, with an average gain of eight years. The Russian Federation would gain more than 10 years. In contrast, health gains from reducing child and maternal mortality would be much more modest: reaching the levels prescribed by the MDGs would raise life expectancy at birth in the region by only 0.7–1.2 years, while reaching European Union levels would result in 0.9–2.0 years of gain.

According to the World Bank report, the greatest potential contributor to health gains in this region would be the reduction of deaths from cardiovascular diseases. The figure below shows the estimated impact of two scenarios: (1) reduction of infant, child and maternal mortality rates to the MDG levels; (2) reduction of mortality from cardiovascular diseases and external causes of death (injuries, violence and poisoning) to European Union levels, while keeping infant, child, and maternal mortality rates constant (*42*).

The impact of two scenarios on life expectancy in eastern Europe and the former Soviet Union

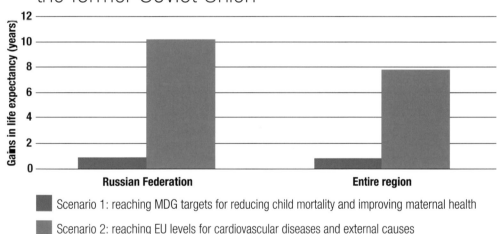

Scenario 1: reaching MDG targets for reducing child mortality and improving maternal health

Scenario 2: reaching EU levels for cardiovascular diseases and external causes

Chronic disease prevention and control can no longer be ignored as an important means of poverty reduction, and more generally, economic development. Investment in chronic disease prevention programmes is essential for many low and middle income countries struggling to reduce poverty. Several countries have adapted the MDG targets and indicators to include chronic diseases. These adaptations are needed to achieve Goal 6, on combating HIV/AIDS, malaria and other diseases, and a selection are featured in the table on the next page.

Adaptations to Millennium Development Goal 6: Combat HIV/AIDS, malaria and other diseases

Czech Republic
New target added: reduce morbidity and mortality caused by main chronic diseases

Mauritius
New target added: have halted by 2015, and begun to reverse, the incidence of noncommunicable diseases such as diabetes, hypertension, high cholesterol, cancer, etc.

Poland
New target added: reduce premature adult mortality by 25% by 2010 (primarily due to tobacco and alcohol use, and unhealthy diet)

Slovakia
New target added: decrease the spread of cancers to the level of EU countries and decrease the prevalence of respiratory diseases

Thailand
New indicators added: heart disease prevalence and death rates

Importance of chronic disease noted in country MDG reports

Hungary
Tobacco use, cardiovascular disease and cancer are noted as primary contributors to premature mortality

Indonesia
Tobacco use is reported as a major contributor to ill health, accounting for a large proportion of the total disease burden

Jordan
Cardiovascular disease and cancer are noted as additional health problems

Lithuania
Cardiovascular disease and cancer are noted as the leading causes of death

CONCLUSION

This chapter has illustrated some of the relationships between chronic diseases and poverty. As a country develops economically, chronic disease risks may first increase among the wealthy but soon concentrate among the poor. In almost all countries poverty increases the risk of developing a chronic disease, and everywhere increases the chances of developing complications and dying prematurely. Chronic diseases can cause individuals and families to fall into poverty and create a downward spiral of worsening poverty and disease. But the impact is not only on individuals and their families. As the next chapter shows, chronic diseases also hinder the macroeconomic development of many countries.

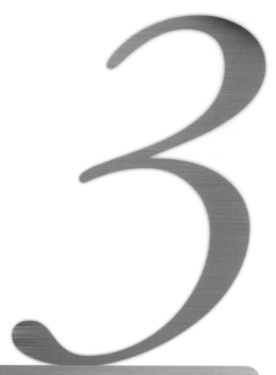

3 The economic impact of chronic diseases

>> **Chronic diseases are a major cost and a profound economic burden to individuals, their families, health systems and societies**

>> **These costs will increase without the implementation of effective interventions**

>> **Investment in interventions to control the burden of chronic diseases will bring appreciable economic benefits**

This chapter presents estimates of the economic impact of selected chronic diseases – heart disease, stroke and diabetes – using three approaches. First, cost of illness studies are summarized. Second, the impact of premature mortality from these diseases on the national income of selected countries is estimated. Third, the "full costs" or welfare losses of chronic disease are assessed. Finally, the potential gains to the economies of these countries – were the global goal to be achieved – are estimated.

MEASURING THE COSTS OF CHRONIC DISEASES

Chronic diseases have an impact on national economies in a number of direct and indirect ways. They reduce the quantity and productivity of labour. In agricultural communities, the pattern of planting crops may change and the timing of critical activities, such as planting or harvesting, can be delayed. Medical expenses deplete savings and investment, including investment in the education of children. All these factors reduce the earning potential of individuals and households, and affect the national economy. An important component of the socioeconomic impact of chronic diseases is, therefore, the effect on income or earnings at the household level, and national income or gross domestic product at the national level.

The cost of chronic disease can be estimated in three ways: the accounting cost of illness method; economic growth models, which estimate the impact of chronic diseases on national income through variables such as labour supply and savings; and the full-income method, which attempts to measure the welfare losses associated with ill-health in money terms. The majority of published studies on the costs of chronic diseases have employed the accounting cost method. Very few have used economic growth and full-income models. Estimates from all methods vary in degree of completeness and are subject to a wide range of interpretations. Estimates from the economic growth approach give the lowest estimates, the full-income approach gives the highest estimates, while cost of illness estimates fall between the two. A summary of the methods used in this chapter is given in Annex 4 (a more detailed description is available at http://www.who.int/chp/chronic_disease_report/en/, including a full list of references).

COST OF ILLNESS STUDIES

The direct costs of health-care resources and non-medical goods and services consumed in the treatment of chronic diseases are enormous. Estimates vary by country, by year and for the same year in any country, reflecting differences in the level of health-care access and delivery, the financing systems of the countries, and methodological variations (43–49).

In the United States, the estimated total health-care costs resulting from heart disease increased from US$ 298.2 billion in 2000, to US$ 329.2 billion in 2001 and US$ 351.8 billion in 2002 (46). The estimated 2 million stroke cases in the United States in 1996 cost the health-care system US$ 8.3 billion, and caused 5.2 million work days to be lost. In the United Kingdom, heart disease cost the health-care system £1.7 billion (approximately US$ 3 billion) in 1999: £2.4 billion (approximately US$ 4.3 billion) in informal care and £2.9 billion (approximately US$ 5.2 billion) in loss of productivity (*49*). Stroke cost the National Health Service £15 303 (approximately US$ 27 306) over five years for every person who experienced a stroke, rising to £29 405 (approximately US$ 52 470) (2001/2002 prices) if informal care is included. Heart disease alone cost 6% of National Health Service revenue at 1994–95 prices (*48*). In Australia, stroke is estimated to be responsible for about 2% of the country's total attributable direct health-care costs (*50–52*).

RISK FACTORS IMPOSE AN ECONOMIC BURDEN ON SOCIETY

Overlapping somewhat with these estimates, obesity has been reported to account for approximately 5% of national health expenditure in the United States, and from 2% to 3.5% in other countries (see figure below). Some studies have highlighted effects of the burden of obesity from other perspectives, for example on health insurance plans, as well as the impact of obesity on future disease risks and associated medical care costs.

Proportion of national health expenditure attributable to obesity in selected countries

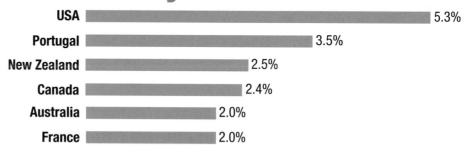

USA	5.3%
Portugal	3.5%
New Zealand	2.5%
Canada	2.4%
Australia	2.0%
France	2.0%

Source: Adapted from Thomson D, Wolf AM, 2001 (*53*).

The direct health expenditures attributable to physical inactivity have been estimated at approximately 2.5% of health expenditure in Canada and the United States (*54*). In 1999, the World Bank estimated that tobacco-related health care accounts for between 6% and 15% of all annual health-care costs (*55, 56*) and between 0.1% and 1.1% of GDP (*57*) in high income countries.

A large proportion of these costs is avoidable and shows the extent of the savings that could be made. Evidence suggests that a modest reduction in the prevalence of certain chronic disease risk factors could result in substantial health gains and cost savings. For instance, a Norwegian study estimated that savings of US$ 188 million from averted heart disease and stroke over 25 years would result from lowering the population blood pressure level by 2 mmHg, by means of a reduction in salt intake (58). A Canadian study estimated that a 10% reduction in the prevalence of physical inactivity could reduce direct health-care expenditures by C$ 150 million (approximately US$ 124 million) in a year. It is clear that chronic diseases and their risk factors impose significant costs on the health systems of countries where people have good access to care.

MACROECONOMIC CONSEQUENCES OF CHRONIC DISEASES

In addition to measuring direct costs, cost of illness studies traditionally also measure indirect costs or the lost production associated with the disease. This is usually rather simplistically assumed to be the total time lost through premature death and illness (mostly self-reported lost days, which overestimate true lost days) multiplied by a wage rate, and sometimes accounting for unemployment. The sums of direct and indirect costs are then assumed to be the loss of GDP. This is incorrect for a variety of reasons. A more appropriate way of considering the GDP cost of chronic diseases is used in this report.

The Solow economic growth model was applied under conservative assumptions of projected chronic disease mortality and a combination of other economic parameters (details are provided in Annex 4). The model was calibrated for each country for 2002, and then GDP was projected to 2015. Estimates of variations in output with respect to labour were taken from previous growth models, some of which did not have access to the exact size of the labour force, so the total population aged 15–64 years was used. To be consistent, the size of the working-age population has also been used in the estimates.

In addition, the impact of direct medical expenditures on growth was captured through the assumption that a certain proportion would be met from savings, which in turn reduces growth. Projections were made of national income with or without mortality and medical expenditures associated with disease, with the difference representing the value of foregone national income. The assumptions used in this chapter are deliberately conservative.

The base estimates presented here show that countries will potentially lose substantial amounts of national income as a result of the impact of deaths from chronic diseases on labour supplies and savings. In 2005, the estimated losses in national income from heart disease, stroke and diabetes (reported in international dollars to account for differences in purchasing power between countries)[1] are 18 billion dollars in China, 11 billion dollars in the Russian Federation, 9 billion dollars in India and 3 billion dollars in Brazil. Similarly, the losses for the United Kingdom, Pakistan, Canada, Nigeria and the United Republic of Tanzania are 1.6 billion, 1.2 billion, 0.5 billion, 0.4 billion, and 0.1 billion international dollars, respectively.

These losses accumulate over time because each year more people die. Estimates for 2015 for the same countries are between approximately three and six times those of 2005. The cumulative and average losses are higher in the larger countries like China, India and the Russian Federation, and are as high as 558 billion international dollars in China.

Projected foregone national income due to heart disease, stroke and diabetes, selected countries, 2005–2015 (billions of constant 1998 international dollars)

	Brazil	Canada	China	India	Nigeria	Pakistan	Russian Federation	United Kingdom	United Republic of Tanzania
Estimated income loss in 2005	2.7	0.5	18.3	8.7	0.4	1.2	11.1	1.6	0.1
Estimated income loss in 2015	9.3	1.5	131.8	54.0	1.5	6.7	66.4	6.4	0.5
Accumulated loss in 2005 value	49.2	8.5	557.7	236.6	7.6	30.7	303.2	32.8	2.5

These losses can be translated into percentage reductions in GDP by comparing what would have happened to GDP in the absence of chronic diseases with what happens in their presence (see figure opposite). In 2005, chronic diseases are estimated to reduce GDP by less than 0.5% in most of the countries, and by 1% in the Russian Federation. By 2015, the percentage reduction in GDP would be over 5% in the Russian

[1] An international dollar is a hypothetical currency that is used as a means of translating and comparing costs from one country to the other using a common reference point, the US dollar. An international dollar has the same purchasing power as the US dollar has in the United States.

Federation and around 1% in the other countries. The absolute loss in dollar terms would be highest in the most populous countries, not unexpectedly, such as India and China. However, the greatest percentage loss would be in the Russian Federation where the cardiovascular disease rates are much greater than in the other countries.

Projected annual reduction in GDP from deaths due to heart disease, stroke and diabetes as proportion of GDP, 2005–2015

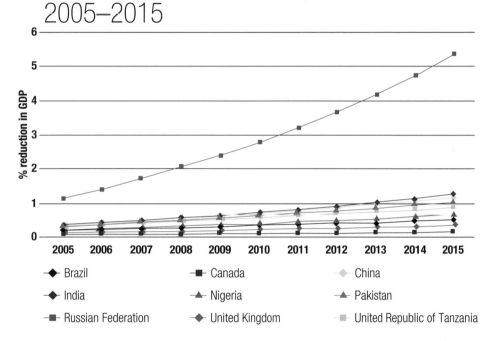

- ◆ Brazil
- ■ Canada
- ◆ China
- ◆ India
- ▲ Nigeria
- ▲ Pakistan
- ■ Russian Federation
- ◆ United Kingdom
- ■ United Republic of Tanzania

ROBUSTNESS OF THE ESTIMATES

Many of the assumptions in this model were tested using sensitivity analysis. The results were robust to even large changes in the majority of the assumptions, including the costs of treatment.

This analysis is exploratory, but seeks to measure the impact of chronic diseases on GDP in a way that is consistent with economic theory. A number of the possible pathways between illness and macroeconomic output were not included, such as the impact on children's education, which could in future be included with exploration of the impact of different functional forms. However, this analysis already provides a more realistic idea of the impact on GDP than traditional methods.

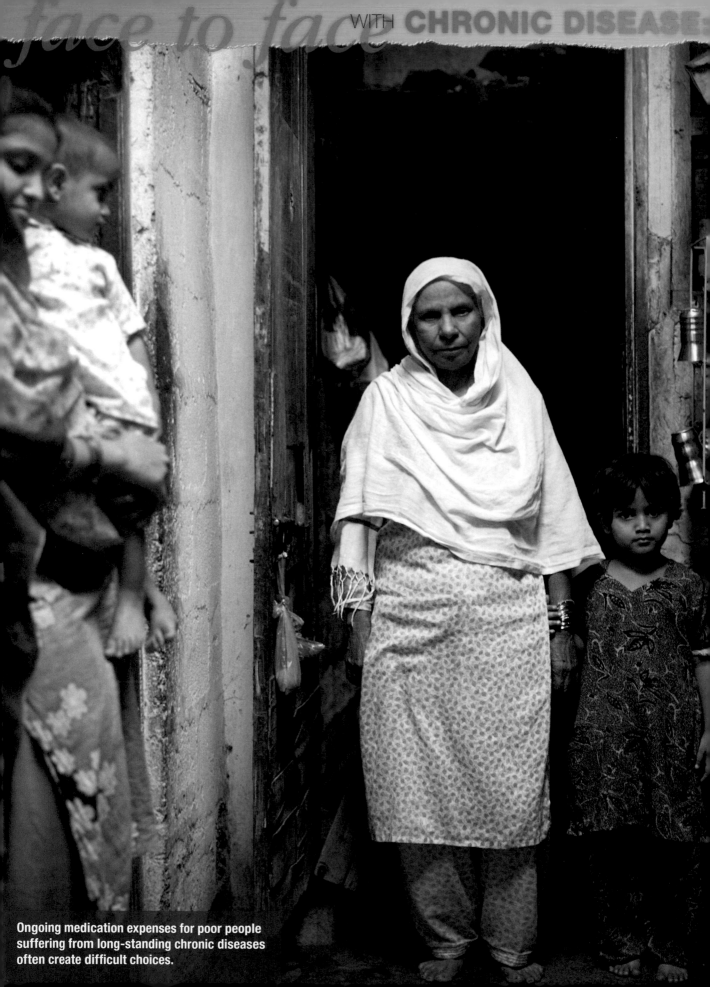

Ongoing medication expenses for poor people suffering from long-standing chronic diseases often create difficult choices.

SHAKEELA BEGUM
FACING A DIRE CHOICE

SHAKEELA BEGUM, NOW 65 YEARS OLD, has been living in fear since she had a heart attack 10 years ago. The fact that she hasn't fully recovered from this ordeal both physically and emotionally makes her life very difficult. "I'm okay when I'm busy, otherwise I keep thinking that I'll have another heart attack," she says with a worried look on her face. "I can't do as much, because I get tired very quickly," she adds.

Name	Shakeela Begum
Age	65
Country	Pakistan
Diagnosis	Heart disease

Like many women her age, Shakeela leads a rather sedentary life in the Karachi home she shares with family. She spends most of her time cleaning and looking after her grandchildren and rarely leaves the house other than for food and medication. "I prefer going to the nearby pharmacy, even if it costs more, than going to the hospital and waiting in line for hours to get my medication," she explains. The downside to this alternative is that, for financial reasons, Shakeela is not buying a sufficient amount of medication and therefore not taking the prescribed dose. "I know I should be taking my medication every day but this way I can also save some money for my grandchildren — they are young and have a future," she argues.

81

THE FULL COSTS OF CHRONIC DISEASES FOR COUNTRIES

In the previous section, the impact of deaths due to chronic diseases on national income was estimated for the selected countries by examining the known relationship between savings, capital stocks and labour availability. The estimated loss of GDP from chronic diseases is just that – the loss of GDP – and does not include the value that people place on losses (or gains) in health. People also value health for its own sake, and suffer welfare losses from poor health and from the death of loved ones.

Recent work has developed an approach called the full-income method that seeks to value the health gains (and by extension, health losses) in monetary terms. These estimates are regarded as changes in economic welfare. Disease and deaths will result in losses to welfare which is greater than the loss of income, and may be regarded as full costs. This section estimates the value of the welfare losses associated with chronic disease deaths using this approach.

Full-income losses due to heart disease, stroke and diabetes in 2005 compared with 2015 estimates

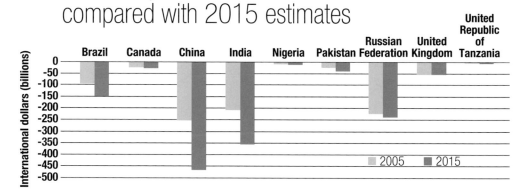

Here, only the mortality associated with heart disease, stroke and diabetes is valued. Following recent suggestions in the literature, the welfare value of a lost life was assumed to be 100 times GDP per capita. Estimates of welfare losses run into billions of dollars for all countries (see figure above), and increase annually as the cumulative toll of mortality increases. Variations across countries are driven by differences in the total number of deaths from these causes and levels of GDP per capita. In Brazil, China, India and the Russian Federation losses are more than a trillion dollars because of the large number of deaths, whereas Canada and the United Kingdom experience lower welfare losses because of fewer deaths from cardiovascular disease in total.

The converse is that these figures could be considered to be potential welfare gains if chronic diseases in these countries were successfully reduced. These gains are clearly much higher than the gains in GDP estimated in the previous section because of the fact that welfare encompasses much more than narrow economic benefits. The numbers should be interpreted with caution, because the approach is not yet well accepted; however, it provides an upper limit for the cost estimates.

ECONOMIC IMPACT OF ACHIEVING THE GLOBAL GOAL IN COUNTRIES

The global goal described in Part One of this report proposes a target of an additional 2% annual reduction in projected chronic disease death rates between 2005 and 2015. This corresponds to the prevention of 36 million premature deaths over the next 10 years. Some 17 million of these prevented deaths would occur in people under 70 years of age.

To estimate the potential economic gain were this scenario to be achieved, the growth model was used, and the loss in national income given the global goal scenario was compared with the loss that would occur given the business-as-usual situation discussed previously.

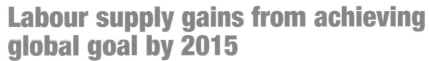

Labour supply gains from achieving global goal by 2015

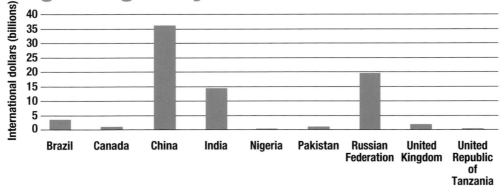

The averted deaths would translate into substantial labour supply gains. This in turn would translate to an accumulated gain in income of over 36 billion dollars in China, 15 billion dollars in India and 20 billion dollars in the Russian Federation over the next 10 years (see figure above).

CONCLUSION

The estimates arrived at by the different methods used here vary – but all indicate that chronic diseases place a grave economic burden on countries, and that this burden will increase if no action is taken. The evidence is clear that action is urgently needed to avoid an adverse impact on national economic development. The cost of achieving the global goal has not been estimated here, although Part Three will show that simple, well-applied policies and interventions targeted at the prevention and control of chronic diseases are cost-effective and affordable.

REFERENCES

1. *The world health report 2001 – Mental health: new understanding, new hope.* Geneva, World Health Organization, 2001.

2. Barker DJ. The developmental origins of chronic adult disease. *Acta Paediatrica Supplement*, 2004, 93:26–33.

3. Pinhas-Hamiel O, Zeitler P. The global spread of type 2 diabetes mellitus in children and adolescents. *Journal of Pediatrics*, 2005, 146:693–700.

4. Ezzati M, Vander Hoorn S, Lawes CM, Leach R, James WP, Lopez AD et al. Rethinking the "diseases of affluence" paradigm: global patterns of nutritional risks in relation to economic development. *PLoS Medicine*, 2005, 2(5):e133.

5. Ezzati M, Lopez AD, Rodgers A, Murray CJL, eds. *Comparative quantification of health risks: global and regional burden of disease attributable to selected major risk factors.* Geneva, World Health Organization, 2004.

6. World Health Organization. *WHO Global InfoBase online* (http://www.who.int/ncd_surveillance/infobase/web/InfoBaseCommon/, accessed 19 July 2005).

7. *The World Health Report 2002 – Reducing risks, promoting healthy life.* Geneva, World Health Organization, 2002.

8. Zatonski WA, Willett WC. *Dramatic decline in coronary heart disease mortality in Poland. Second look* (unpublished manuscript).

9. Capewell S, Beaglehole R, Sessen M, McMurray J. Explanation for the decline in coronary heart disease mortality rates in Auckland, New Zealand, between 1982 and 1993. *Circulation*, 2000, 102:1511–1516.

10. Unal B, Critchley JA, Capewell S. Explaining the decline in coronary heart disease mortality in England and Wales between 1981 and 2000. *Circulation*, 2004, 109:1101–1107.

11. Critchley JA, Capewell S, Unal B. Life-years gained from coronary heart disease mortality reduction in Scotland: prevention or treatment? *Journal of Clinical Epidemiology*, 2003, 56:583–90.

12. Strong K, Mathers C, Leeder S, Beaglehole R. Preventing chronic diseases: how many lives can we save? *Lancet* (in press), 2005.

13. Sachs JD. *The end of poverty.* New York, NY, Penguin Press, 2005.

14. Marmot M. *Status syndrome.* London, Bloomsbury, 2004.

15. Gwatkin DR, Bhuiya A, Victora CG. Making health systems more equitable. *Lancet*, 2004, 364:1273–1280.

16. Machenbach JP, Bos V, Andersen O, Cardano M, Costa G, Harding S et al. Widening socioeconomic inequalities in mortality in six Western European countries. *International Journal of Epidemiology*, 2003, 32:830–837.

17. Bartley M, Fitzpatrick R, Firth D, Marmot M. Social distribution of cardiovascular disease risk factors: change among men in England 1984-1993. *Journal of Epidemiology and Community Health*, 2000, 54:806–814.

18. Yu Z, Nissinen A, Vartiainen E, Song G, Guo Z, Zheng G et al. Associations between socioeconomic status and cardiovascular risk factors in an urban population in China. *Bulletin of the World Health Organization*, 2000, 78:1296–1305.

19. Bovet P, Ross AG, Gervasoni JP, Mkamba M, Mtasiwa DM, Lengeler C et al. Distribution of blood pressure, body mass index and smoking habits in the urban population of Dar es Salaam, Tanzania, and associations with socioeconomic status. *International Journal of Epidemiology*, 2002, 31:240–247.

20. Drewnowski A. Obesity and the food environment: dietary energy density and diet costs. *American Journal of Preventive Medicine*, 2004, 27(3 Suppl.):154–162.

21. Stronks K, Van de Mheen HD, Mackenbach JP. A higher prevalence of health problems in low income groups: does it reflect relative deprivation? *Journal of Epidemiology and Community Health*, 1998, 52:548–557.

22. Sundquist K, Malmstrom M, Johansson SE. Neighbourhood deprivation and incidence of coronary heart disease: a multilevel study of 2.6 million women and men in Sweden. *Journal of Epidemiology and Community Health*, 2004, 58:71–77.

23. Goddard M, Smith P. *Equity of access to health care.* York, University of York, 1998.

24. Lorant V, Boland B, Humblet P, Deliege D. Equity in prevention and health care. *Journal of Epidemiology and Community Health*, 2002, 56:510–516.

25. Heisler M, Langa KM, Eby EL, Fendrick AM, Kabeto MU, Piette JD. The health effects of restricting prescription medication use because of cost. *Medical Care*, 2004, 42:626–634.

26. Alberts M, Olwagen R, Molaba CJ, Choma S. *Socio-economic status and the diagnosis, treatment and control of hypertension in the Dikgale Field Site, South Africa.* INDEPTH Network Working Paper Series No. 2, 2005 (http://www.indepth-network.org/publications/zindpubs/wpseries/wpseries.htm, accessed 15 July 2005).

27. *Women of South-East Asia: a health profile.* New Delhi, World Health Organization Regional Office for South-East Asia, 2000 (http://w3.whosea.org/EN/Section13/Section390/Section1376_5513.htm, accessed 12 July 2005).

28. Lewallen S, Courtright P. Gender and use of cataract surgical services in developing countries. *Bulletin of the World Health Organization*, 2002, 80:300–303.

29. Zohoori N, Blanchette D, Popkin B. *Monitoring health conditions in the Russian Federation. The Russia Longitudinal Monitoring Survey 1992-2002.* Report submitted to the US Agency for International Development. Chapel Hill, NC, Carolina Population Center, University of North Carolina at Chapel Hill, 2003.

30. Henry-Lee A, Yearwood A. *Protecting the poor and the medically indigent under health insurance: a case study in Jamaica.* Bethesda, MD, Partnership for Health Reform Project and Abt Associates, 1999.

31. Shobhana R, Rama RP, Lavanya A, Williams R, Vijay V, Ramachandran A. Expenditure on health care incurred by diabetic subjects in a developing country – a study from southern India. *Diabetes Research and Clinical Practice*, 2000, 48:37–42.

32. Narayan D, Chambers R, Shah M, Petesch P. *Voices of the poor crying out for change*. New York, NY, Oxford University Press for the World Bank, 2000.

33. Hulme D, Shepherd A. Conceptualizing chronic poverty. *World Development*, 2003, 31:403–423.

34. Liu Y, Keqin R, Hsiao W. Medical expenditure and rural impoverishment in China. *Journal of Health, Population and Nutrition*, 2003, 21:216–222.

35. Kraut A, Walld R, Tate R, Mustard C. Impact of diabetes on employment and income in Manitoba, Canada. *Diabetes Care*, 2001, 24:64–68.

36. Kochar A. Ill-health, savings and portfolio choices in developing countries. *Journal of Developing Economics*, 2004, 73:257–285.

37. *Tobacco and poverty: a vicious circle*. Geneva, World Health Organization, 2004 (WHO/NMH/TFI/04.01).

38. Bonu S, Rani M, Peters DH, Jha P, Nguyen SN. Does use of tobacco or alcohol contribute to impoverishment from hospitalization costs in India? *Health Policy and Planning*, 2005, 20:41–49.

39. Suhrcke M, Rocco L, Urban D, McKee M, Mazzuco S, Steinherr A. *Economic consequences of non-communicable disease and injuries in Russian Federation* [draft]. Venice, World Health Organization European Office for Investment for Health and Development, 2005.

40. Roy NC, Kane T, Barket-e-Khuda. Socioeconomic and health implications of adults deaths in families of rural Bangladesh. *Journal of Health, Population and Nutrition*, 2001, 19:291–300.

41. *Health and the Millennium Development Goals*. Geneva, World Health Organization, 2005.

42. Rechel B, Shapo L, McKee M. *Millennium Development Goals for health in Europe and Central Asia: relevance and policy implications*. Washington, DC, World Bank, 2004.

43. Cohen JW, Krauss NA. Spending and service use among people with the fifteen most costly medical conditions, 1997. *Health Affairs*, 2003, 22:129–138.

44. Druss BG, Marcus SC, Olfson M, Tanielian T, Elinson L, Pincus HA. Comparing the national economic burden of five chronic conditions. *Health Affairs,* 2001, 20:233–241.

45. Druss BG, Marcus SC, Olfson M, Pincus HA. The most expensive medical conditions in America. *Health Affairs*, 2002, 21:105–111.

46. *Heart disease and stroke statistics – 2001 update*. Dallas, TX, American Heart Association, 2001.

47. Russell MW, Huse DM, Drowns S, Hamel EC, Hartz SC. Direct medical costs of coronary artery disease in the United States. *American Journal of Cardiology*, 1998. 81:1110–1115.

48. Currie CJ, Morgan CL, Peters JR. Patterns and costs of hospital care for coronary heart disease related and not related to diabetes. *Heart*, 1997, 78:544–549.

49. Liu JL, Maniadakis N, Gray A, Rayner M. The economic burden of coronary heart disease in the UK. *Heart*, 2002, 88:597–603.

50. *Preliminary estimates: Disease Costs and Impact Study (DCIS)*. Canberra, Australian Institute of Health and Welfare/Centre for Health Program Evaluation, 1995.

51. Waters A-M, Armstrong T, Senes-Ferrari S. *Medical care of cardiovascular disease in Australia*. Canberra, Australian Institute of Health and Welfare, 1998.

52. Dewey HM, Thrift AG, Mihalopoulos C, Carter R, Macdonell RA, McNeil JJ et al. Cost of stroke in Australia from a societal perspective: results from the North East Melbourne Stroke Incidence Study (NEMESIS). *Stroke*, 2001, 32:2409–2416.

53. Thompson D, Wolf AM. The medical-care cost burden of obesity. *Obesity Reviews*, 2001, 2:189–197.

54. Katzmarzyk PT, Janssen I. The economic costs associated with physical inactivity and obesity in Canada: an update. *Canadian Journal of Applied Physiology,* 2004, 29:90–115.

55. *Curbing the epidemic: governments and the economics of tobacco control.* Washington, DC, World Bank, 1999.

56. Lightwood JM, Collins D, Lapsley H, Novotny T. Estimating the costs of tobacco use. In: Jha P, Chaloupka F, eds. *Tobacco control in developing countries.* Oxford, Oxford University Press, 2000.

57. Hodgson TA. Cigarette smoking and lifetime medical expenditures. *The Milbank Quarterly,* 1992, 70:81–125.

58. Selmer RM, Kristiansen IS, Haglerod A, Graff-Iversen S, Larsen HK, Meyer HE et al. Cost and health consequences of reducing the population intake of salt. *Journal of Epidemiology and Community Health*, 2000, 54:697–702.

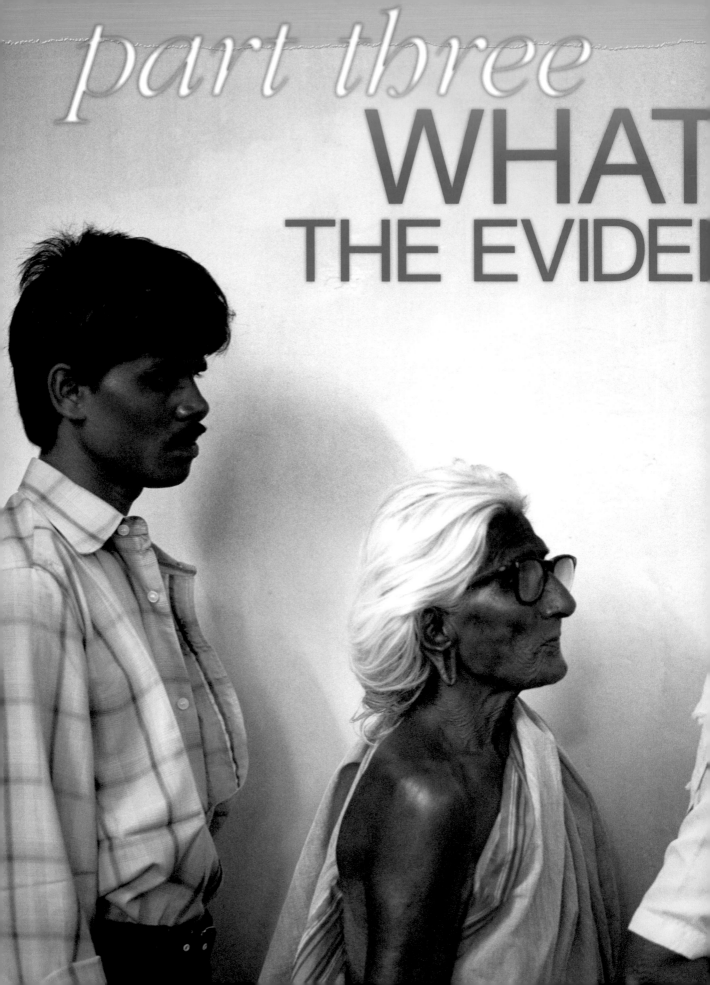

part three

WHAT

THE EVIDE

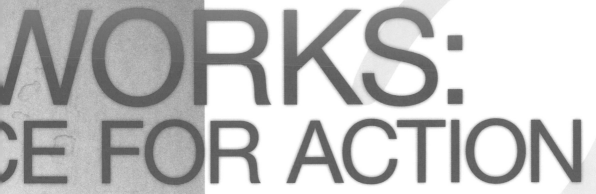

WORKS:
CE FOR ACTION

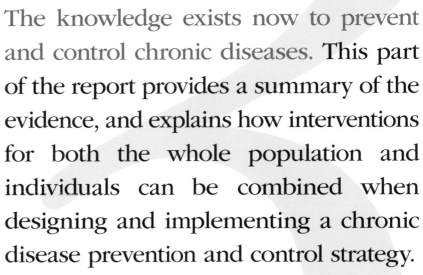

The knowledge exists now to prevent and control chronic diseases. This part of the report provides a summary of the evidence, and explains how interventions for both the whole population and individuals can be combined when designing and implementing a chronic disease prevention and control strategy.

key messages

» **Chronic diseases can be prevented and controlled using available knowledge**

» **Comprehensive and integrated action is required**

face to face
WITH **CHRONIC DISEASE**

MILTON PAULO FLORET FRANZOLIN
"I don't want to be a victim but a fighter"
94

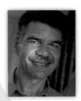

ZAHIDA BIBI
Suffering from preventable complications
114

89

1 A strategy to achieve rapid results

Population-wide approaches seek to reduce the risks throughout the entire population. They address the causes rather than the consequences of chronic diseases and are central to attempts to prevent the emergence of future epidemics. Small reductions in the exposure of the population to risk factors such as tobacco use, unhealthy diet and physical inactivity lead to population-level reductions in cholesterol, blood pressure, blood glucose and body weight. More fundamentally, interventions are also required to address the underlying determinants of chronic disease, as described in Part Two.

>> **Rapid health gains can be achieved with comprehensive and integrated action**

>> **In this way, many countries and regions have already successfully curbed chronic diseases**

Interventions for individuals focus on people who are at high risk and those with established chronic disease. These interventions reduce the risk of developing chronic disease, reduce complications, and improve quality of life.

Population-wide and individual approaches are complementary. They should be combined as part of a comprehensive strategy that serves the needs of the entire population and has an impact at the individual, community and national levels. Comprehensive approaches should also be integrated: covering all the major risk factors and cutting across specific diseases.

RAPID HEALTH GAINS CAN BE ACHIEVED

It is not necessary to wait decades to reap the benefits of prevention and control activities. Risk factor reduction can lead to surprisingly rapid health gains, at both population and individual levels. This can be observed through national trends (in Finland and Poland, for example, as described on page 93), sub-national epidemiological data and clinical trials.

In the case of tobacco control, the impact of proactive policies and programmes is almost immediate. The implementation of tobacco-free policies leads to quick decreases in tobacco use, rates of cardiovascular disease, and hospitalizations from myocardial infarction.

Improving diet and physical activity can prevent type 2 diabetes among those at high risk in a very short space of time. In China, Finland and the USA, for example, study participants have significantly improved their diet and/or physical activity, and shown improved levels of blood pressure, blood glucose, cholesterol and triglycerides as quickly as one year after starting a programme, with improvements continuing for at least six years. The incidence of diabetes was reduced by almost 60% in both Finland and the USA, and by over 30% in China (1–3).

Lowering a person's serum cholesterol concentration results in quick and substantial protection from heart disease. Benefits are related to age: a 10% reduction in serum cholesterol in men aged 40 can result in a 50% reduction in heart disease, while at age 70 there is on average a 20% reduction. Benefits can be realized quickly – after two years – with full benefits coming after five years (4).

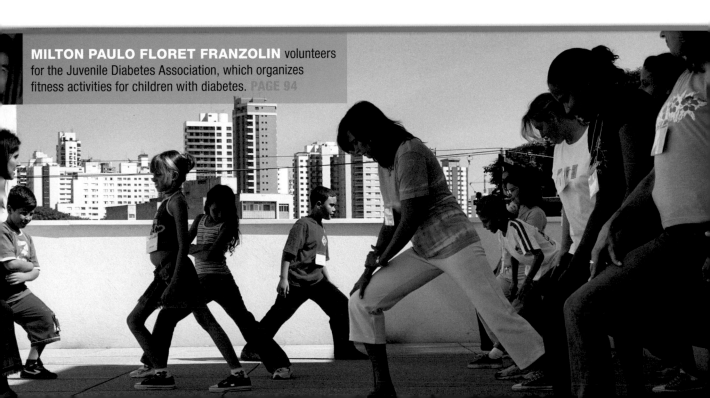

MILTON PAULO FLORET FRANZOLIN volunteers for the Juvenile Diabetes Association, which organizes fitness activities for children with diabetes. PAGE 94

REGIONAL AND NATIONAL SUCCESS STORIES

Death rates from the major chronic diseases, especially cardiovascular diseases, have decreased dramatically over the past three decades in several countries in which effective programmes have been introduced, but have increased in countries where no such programmes exist. While Australia, Canada, the United Kingdom and the United States, for example, have achieved steady declines in heart disease death rates, the rates in other countries, such as Brazil and the Russian Federation, have remained the same or increased (see figure below).

How were these dramatic results achieved? Initial reductions occurred partly as a result of the diffusion of health-related information to the general population. Later, integrated and comprehensive approaches were successfully implemented. These approaches have been used to reduce chronic disease death rates in many countries, demonstrating the feasibility of achieving more widespread success.

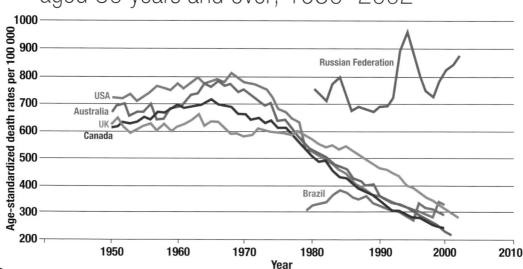

Heart disease death rates among men aged 30 years and over, 1950–2002

A DRAMATIC REDUCTION IN THE DEATH RATE IN POLAND

Between 1960 and 1990, Poland experienced a serious increase in death rates from heart disease among young and middle-aged men and women. Unexpectedly, beginning with political and economic changes in 1991, this trend sharply reversed. In people aged between 20 and 44 years, the decline in death rates averaged 10% annually, while in those aged between 45 and 64 years, the annual rate of decline was 6.7%. This was one of the most dramatic rates of decline ever seen in Europe, although similar declines have since occurred in other countries in eastern Europe.

Poland's results have been attributed principally to the replacement of dietary saturated fat with polyunsaturated fat. Vegetable fat and oil consumption increased (primarily in the form of rape-seed and soybean oil products), while animal fat consumption, mainly butter, declined. These trends were associated with the removal of price subsidies on butter and the availability of cheaper vegetable oils. Other factors contributing to the decline include increased fruit consumption and decreased tobacco use (but only in men). Improvements in medical treatment contributed little, if at all, to the decline in death rates (5, 6).

REDUCING DEATH RATES FROM HEART DISEASE IN FINLAND

In the 1970s, Finland had the world's highest death rate from cardiovascular disease. This was largely a result of widespread and heavy tobacco use, high-fat diet and low vegetable intake. In response to local concerns, a large-scale community-based intervention was organized, involving consumers, schools, and social and health services. It included legislation banning tobacco advertising, the introduction of low-fat dairy and vegetable oil products, changes in farmers' payment schemes (linking payment for milk to protein rather than fat content), and incentives for communities achieving the greatest cholesterol reduction.

Death rates from heart disease in men have been reduced by at least 65%, and lung cancer death rates in men have also fallen. Greatly reduced cardiovascular and cancer mortality has led to greater life expectancy – approximately seven years for men and six years for women (7).

Heart disease and lung cancer death rates among men aged 30 years and over in Finland

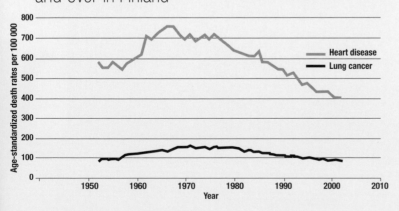

ELIMINATING TRACHOMA IN MOROCCO

Morocco is on track to achieve the elimination of blinding trachoma by 2006. This success has resulted from a combination of high-level political commitment, partnerships and community participation in prevention and control efforts.

Trachoma is a chronic disease with an infectious origin that results in irreversible blindness if untreated. It was common in Morocco in the 1970s and 1980s. A national assessment in the early 1990s found that despite existing activities, the disease was still blinding the poor citizens of five provinces who were not yet benefiting from the development of services and infrastructure seen elsewhere. An integrated programme backed by the King of Morocco and Ministry of Health officials was implemented with external partners. The programme included provision of surgical services to stop the progression of blindness, health promotion and environmental measures to prevent infection, and treatment with antibiotics in trachoma-endemic areas.

As a result, in the last 10 years more than 80 000 people have had progression of blindness prevented through surgery; more than 700 000 people were treated with antibiotics; over 40 000 sessions per year were organized to educate communities about primary prevention; some 8000 women per year received literacy education; and more than 80% of rural villages gained access to water points (from 14% in 1990).

In rural disease-endemic areas, trachoma elimination has also been the entry point for introducing a surveillance system, which is now used for chronic diseases generally, developing the primary health care system, and enhancing eye and other health care interventions. Trachoma surgery is integrated with cataract services and dental care. Villages have also received support for the development of income-generating activities, with some of the revenue supporting health promotion and health service provision for children and the elderly.

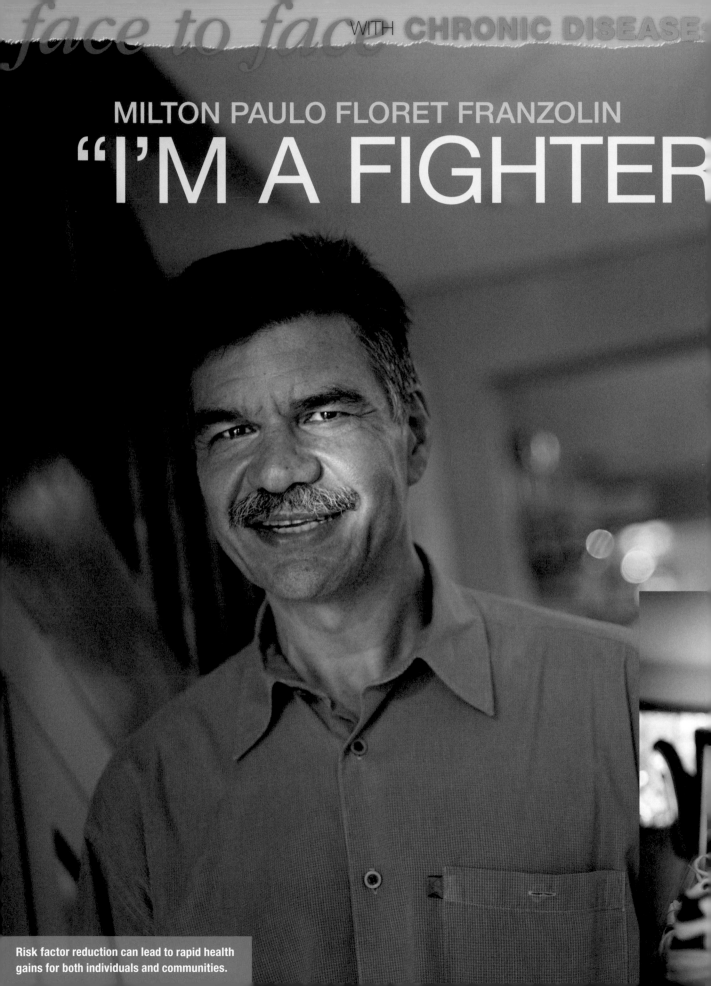

MILTON PAULO FLORET FRANZOLIN

"I'M A FIGHTER

Risk factor reduction can lead to rapid health gains for both individuals and communities.

NOT A VICTIM"

BRAZIL

Name	Milton Franzolin
Age	52
Country	Brazil
Diagnosis	Diabetes

MILTON PAULO FLORET FRANZOLIN has always been a sportsman. He trains for marathons and plays squash twice a week. In 2003, at the age of 50, he was diagnosed with diabetes following his yearly medical check-up. "At first I was revolted and didn't understand how I'd become ill," he says. "My frustration didn't last for long, I didn't want to be a victim but rather, a fighter."

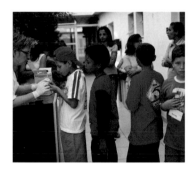

Ironically, Milton had been working as a volunteer with the Juvenile Diabetes Association of São Paulo for two years before being diagnosed with the disease. He had been developing a programme which

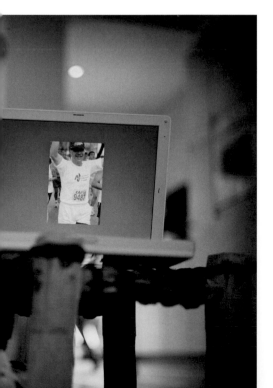

enables children with diabetes to exercise safely. "My goal is to prove that you can live a normal life and be physically competitive even if you have diabetes," he explains.

More than ever, Milton is convinced that awareness is crucial to maintaining health and avoiding complications. "Treatment for diabetes may have improved lately but it is still difficult for poorer people living with the disease to have access to the information they need," he says.

Milton now believes that being diagnosed with diabetes is the best thing that ever happened to him as he feels deeply that he's making a difference through his actions. "It is a privilege and great feeling to be able to influence people's lives, especially those of youngsters," he adds. He encourages others to do the same.

2 Review of effective interventions

Comprehensive and integrated action is the means to prevent and control chronic diseases. This chapter describes and gives examples of the types of interventions, for the whole population or for individuals, that will enable countries to achieve major reductions in premature chronic disease deaths. The chapter outlines the evidence showing that chronic diseases can be prevented and controlled using available knowledge. Moreover, it shows that the solutions are not only effective but can be highly cost-effective even in settings with few resources.

>> **A small shift in the average population levels of several risk factors can lead to a large reduction of the burden of chronic diseases**

>> **Population-wide approaches form the central strategy for preventing chronic disease epidemics, but should be combined with interventions for individuals**

>> **Many interventions are not only effective but are also suitable for resource-constrained settings**

LAWS AND REGULATIONS

National and local legislation, regulations, ordinances, international laws and treaties and other legal frameworks are fundamental elements of effective public health policy and practice. Historically, laws have played a crucial role in some of the greatest achievements in public health such as environmental control laws, seat-belt laws, warnings on cigarette packs and other tobacco control measures, and water fluoridation to reduce dental caries.

Current laws relating to chronic disease have proved to be an effective and central component of comprehensive prevention and control strategies. Advertising bans for tobacco products and the reduction of salt in food (whether through voluntary agreement with industry or enforced) are both very cost-effective in all regions, as assessed by the WHO-CHOICE project.[1]

MORE COULD BE DONE

Legal frameworks have been used extensively with regard to tobacco control, although the WHO Framework Convention on Tobacco Control is the only global framework. Legislation and regulations could be used more effectively to reduce the burden of chronic disease, and to protect the rights of people with a chronic disease.

[1] The WHO-CHOICE project analyses the health effects and costs of interventions (see Annex 5). Interventions are grouped into three broad categories: very cost-effective, cost-effective or cost- ineffective. Results presented in this publication represent a sub-set of all the interventions that were studied by the WHO-CHOICE project, and were selected based on their relevance to chronic disease prevention and control, as well as their cost–effectiveness.

SPOTLIGHT
TOBACCO CONTROL IN THE PHILIPPINES

In 1999, the Philippines introduced major changes in tobacco control policies which have contributed to positive changes.

The Philippines Clear Air Act of 1999 identified cigarette smoke as a pollutant and instituted smoke-free indoor air laws. The national law allows designated smoking areas in restaurants and other indoor areas, but some cities have declared all indoor areas to be completely smoke-free. Taxes on cigarettes have also been increased.

The Youth Smoking Cessation Programme in 2003 declared campuses to be smoke-free, improved training for students and teachers, and levied penalties for smoking.

The Tobacco Regulatory Act of 2003 seeks to increase public education measures, ban all tobacco advertising, strengthen warning labels on tobacco products, and prohibit sales to minors.

All programmes have received extensive national and local media coverage. Evidence of the success of this legislation in combination with other interventions can be seen in the significant drop in the number of students who reported being current cigarette smokers or using other tobacco products over the period 2000–2003. The percentage of students who had never smoked but were likely to initiate smoking in the next year also decreased, from 27% in 2000 to 14% in 2003. Among adolescent boys, the percentage of current tobacco smokers declined by around a third, from 33% in 2000 to 22% in 2003. Among adolescent girls, the decline was similar, from 13% in 2000 to 9% in 2003 (8).

SPOTLIGHT
TOBACCO CONTROL IN SINGAPORE

The legislative measures that have been implemented in Singapore to control tobacco use include:

» prohibition of tobacco advertising and promotion;
» restrictions on the sale of tobacco products;
» licensing of sales outlets;
» use of health warnings on cigarette packs;
» restrictions on smoking in public places;
» prohibition of smoking in public by people under the age of 18 years.

Singapore's smoking rate decreased from an overall prevalence rate of 23% in 1977 to 20% in 1984, and to the lowest level ever, 14%, in 1987. However, smoking rates went up to 17% in 1991 and as high as 18% in 1992. This increase stimulated a review of the situation and of the measures in place. Consolidation of the Smoking (Control of Advertisements and Sale of Tobacco) Act in 1993 led to new sections being added. This, together with the 1994 amendments to health warnings to make them more conspicuous and bold, extension of the prohibition of smoking to all air-conditioned offices, and continuing education programmes and progressive increases in taxation, contributed to a second drop in rates, to 17% in 1995 and 15% in 1998 (9).

TAX AND PRICE INTERVENTIONS

Taxation is one policy instrument for reducing the use of tobacco and intake of foods that are high in fat, sugar and salt. Alternatively, subsidies can be used to promote healthy choices or reduce the cost of goods and services that promote physical activity.

Taxation policies can contribute effectively to the reduction of tobacco use and raise revenue for health promotion and disease prevention programmes, as shown in the Australian state of Victoria and subsequently in several other countries, including Thailand.

Price increases encourage people to stop using tobacco products, they prevent others from starting, and they reduce the number of ex-tobacco users who resume the habit. A 10% price increase in tobacco products has been shown to reduce demand by 3–5% in high income countries, and by 8% in low and middle income countries. Young people and the poor are the most responsive to price changes. Taxation of tobacco products is also very cost-effective (as assessed by the WHO-CHOICE project).

Prices affect food choices and consumption patterns, and food and drink taxes also have the potential to generate revenue which can be earmarked for diet, activity and obesity-prevention initiatives.

In some countries, higher prices have been shown to reduce consumption of soft drinks. In Zambia, for example, sales of branded soft drinks dropped dramatically after prices rose. Alternatively, subsidies can encourage healthier food choices. Studies have shown, for example, that price subsidies in schools and in workplaces increase fruit and vegetable consumption.

SPOTLIGHT
TOBACCO TAXATION IN SOUTH AFRICA

In 1994, the Government of South Africa announced that it would increase the tax on tobacco products to 50% of the retail price. This action has contributed to a doubling of the price of tobacco products over the past decade. Along with other tobacco control interventions, tax increases have contributed to a 33% reduction in tobacco use (see figure below). In addition, government revenue from tobacco taxes has more than doubled (*10*).

Cigarette consumption and retail prices of cigarettes in South Africa, 1961–2001

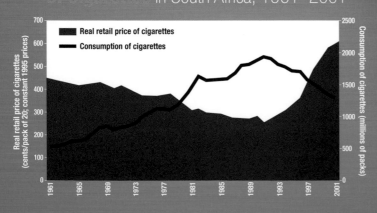

IMPROVING THE BUILT ENVIRONMENT

There are a growing number of examples to show that changing the built environment can lead to increased physical activity. Providing access to exercise facilities, walking and cycle ways, along with compact urban planning, increase the opportunities for, and reduce barriers to, physical activity.

In the Americas, rates of walking and cycling in older neighbourhoods with high population densities, mixed land use, and well-constructed interconnecting footpaths are 30–50% higher than in low-density neighbourhoods typical of suburban sprawl (*11*).

The use of stairs instead of lifts or escalators in public places can be increased by means of signs, posters and music, although the effects are relatively small and short term (*12*).

ADVOCACY

Advocacy interventions use information in deliberate and strategic ways to change decision-makers' perceptions or understanding of an issue and to influence decision-making. They can also shape public perceptions and behaviour and build popular support for policy-making.

A vast array of communication methods is available, the choice depending on the desired outcome. Communication methods range from one-to-one conversations to mass media campaigns and often work better together than individually. They must be selected for their ability to deliver the message effectively and should be tailored to the specific advocacy objective. Common communication methods include information campaigns, publications and web sites, press releases, lobbying and peer-to-peer communication. Health education on cardiovascular risk factors via broadcast and print media has been shown to be very cost-effective in all regions by the WHO-CHOICE project.

SPOTLIGHT
IMPROVING THE BUILT ENVIRONMENT IN COLOMBIA

Over the past 10 years, the city of Bogotá, Colombia, with almost 8 million inhabitants, has made significant progress in promoting physical activity. Safe spaces specifically set aside for leisure activities are now provided, including 128 km of streets exclusively for recreational and sports activities on Sundays and holidays. The city also provides parks, public aerobics classes, a 300 km network of bike paths and a large network of pedestrian-ways. Policies limiting the use of private cars have also been implemented (*13*).

SPOTLIGHT
ADVOCATING FOR PHYSICAL ACTIVITY IN BRAZIL

The Agita São Paulo programme promotes physical activity among the 37 million inhabitants of the state of São Paulo, Brazil. The programme, launched in 1996, organizes "mega-events" such as the Agita Galera Day. In addition to such large-scale events, the programme has over 300 partner institutions, whose main mission is to disseminate the message through their own networks.

Direct costs of the programme are covered largely by the São Paulo State Health Secretariat, with a budget of roughly US$ 150 000, representing an investment of less than US$ 0.5 per inhabitant per year.

Surveys of representative samples of the São Paolo population show that the prevalence of respondents engaging in regular physical activity rose from 55% in 1999 to 60% in 2003. Targeted subgroups showed much more dramatic improvements. For example, of a group of people with high blood pressure and diabetes who received education sessions and personalized advice, there was a reported 96% increase in those who participated in regular physical activity (*14*).

COMMUNITY-BASED INTERVENTIONS

Community-based programmes for chronic disease prevention and control target a specified community. They focus on risk factor reduction, community mobilization and participation.

Integrated community-based programmes aim to reach the general population as well as targeting high-risk and priority populations in schools, workplaces, recreation areas, and religious and health-care settings. They also enable communities to become active participants in decisions concerning their health, and promote simultaneous use of community resources and health services, as well as coordinating different activities by means of partnerships and coalitions.

Successful community-based interventions require partnerships between community organizations, policy-makers, businesses, health providers and community residents. Such interventions for chronic diseases in developed countries have demonstrated considerable potential for effectiveness in developing countries.

Community-based interventions can also be the starting point for national improvement. Finland, featured earlier in this part, is a good example of how community-based programmes, once shown to be successful, can be scaled up to national level (15).

SCHOOL-BASED INTERVENTIONS

School health programmes can be an efficient way of reducing risks among large numbers of children. They vary from one country to another, but almost all include four basic components: health policies, health education, supportive environments and health services. Such programmes often include physical education, nutrition and food services, health promotion for school personnel and outreach to the community.

Many school health programmes focus on preventing the risk factors associated with leading causes of death, disease and disability, such as tobacco, drug and alcohol use, dietary practices, sexual behaviour and physical inactivity.

In comparative studies of public health interventions, the World Bank concluded that school health programmes are highly cost-effective. The annual cost of school health programmes was estimated to be US$ 0.03 per capita in low income countries and US$ 0.06 in middle income countries, respectively, averting 0.1% and 0.4% of the disease burden (16).

SPOTLIGHT
COMMUNITY-BASED PROJECTS IN CHINA

There have been several major community-based projects in China relating to chronic diseases. In China's third largest city, Tianjin, for example, a project was launched in 1984 aimed at reducing chronic disease risk factors at the community level. Activities included training health personnel, health education, health counselling and environmental changes. The nutrition project was integrated into the existing three-level health-care structure in the Tianjin project area without allocation of additional resources. Health workers were trained to increase their knowledge about the relationship between salt intake and blood pressure, and were taught how to give practical advice to patients on this issue.

The project also introduced environmental changes to promote healthy eating habits. Leaflets were distributed door-to-door, and posters and stickers were distributed to food retailers. Special measuring spoons were provided. Low sodium salt was also introduced, and the project cooperated with salt manufacturers and shops to ensure that this salt was available in the intervention area.

An outcome of the study was that residents in the intervention area had significantly better knowledge about salt intake than residents in an area not taking part. In the intervention area, average salt intake was significantly lower in men, and also reduced in women. In addition, there was a significant decrease in systolic blood pressure in the intervention area for both men and women. In contrast, both salt intake and systolic blood pressure increased significantly during the same period in men who did not take part.

In 1995, after comprehensive reviews by the Ministry of Health, Foreign Loan Office and the World Bank, a new project – the World Bank Loan Health VII: China Disease Prevention Project – was undertaken in seven cities, as well as some regions of Yunnan Province, covering a population of 90 million. It included activities in four fields: institutional development and policy reform, human resource development, surveillance and community intervention. Among the outcomes reported was a reduction in the prevalence of male adult cigarette smokers from 59% to 44%. In Beijing there were substantial increases in high blood pressure detection and treatment, and a fall in the death rates for both stroke and heart disease of more than 15% in the last year of the project.

Based on this experience, the Ministry of Health has established a total of 32 demonstration sites for chronic disease prevention and control across the country. Detailed interventions are determined and implemented by local health departments, according to local conditions. Notable outcomes so far have included a reduction in the annual heart disease and stroke deaths in those patients with high blood pressure who were being managed, from 1.6% to 0.8% between 2000 and 2002. In Shenyang, there was a reduction in the prevalence of adult smokers from 29% to 13% between 1997 and 2002 and an increase in the proportion of people participating in planned regular physical activity from 41% to 84% in the same period (*17*).

SPOTLIGHT
SCHOOL-BASED PROGRAMMES IN THE UNITED STATES

The Child and Adolescent Trial for Cardiovascular Health (CATCH) is the largest school-based health study to have been conducted in the United States. It was designed to decrease cardiovascular risk factors in children through:

» modifications to food services to reduce fat consumption;

» smoke-free school policies;

» school health education on cardiovascular risks;

» a complementary family component to educate parents about cardiovascular risks;

» physical education to increase the frequency and intensity of physical activity.

Results demonstrated that children from the intervention schools had lower consumption of total fat and saturated fat, and higher levels of self-reported physical activity, than those from comparison schools. Furthermore, intervention children maintained their results for three years without further interventions.

After five years of follow-up and no further intervention:

» menus from 50% of the former intervention cafeterias met the Eat Smart guidelines for fat compared with 10% of the former control schools;

» student energy expenditure levels and proportion of time spent in moderate-to-vigorous physical activity in the intervention schools had been maintained, although vigorous activity had declined.

These results suggest that changes in the school environment to support health can be maintained over time. Staff training is an important factor in institutionalizing such programmes (18).

VENDING MACHINES

Several interesting school studies have illustrated the ways in which vending machines can be used to promote a healthy diet. A study in the United Kingdom by the Health Education Trust, for example, found that when drink options were increased in school vending machines, even alongside regular options, children chose to drink milk, fruit juices and water. Involving students in decisions related to vending machine choices and the maintenance and location of the machines was important to success (19, 20).

Venice High School in Los Angeles, USA, began offering a variety of waters, 100% juices and soy milk as well as cereal bars to replace the snacks which had previously been sold. After one year, snack sales in the student store were up by over US$ 1000 per month compared with the previous year. Two years after the changes, snack sales per month had roughly doubled (21).

WORKPLACE INTERVENTIONS

Workplace interventions for chronic disease prevention and control are a feasible and often successful means of improving the health of employed adults. Interventions tend to focus on chronic diseases and risk factors that substantially inhibit productivity and incur the most serious health and economic burdens.

Workplace interventions can lead to large gains, both in the short and long term, for employees and employers. Improvements can be seen in worker productivity, reduced levels of absenteeism, and employer cost-saving. These interventions have the added benefit of creating a workplace environment that is health-conscious, providing for easier follow-up with participants.

Programmes that address multiple risk factors for chronic diseases are more successful and improve participation. These programmes allow employees to decide what risk factors they want to improve and define their own goals (22).

Financial rewards, work-related incentives (counting programme time as part of core work hours, for example), discounts on fitness activities, or even simply providing programmes free of charge can increase participation in and adherence to workplace interventions. A comprehensive approach including both policies and programmes, rather than either in isolation, increases the likelihood that employees will participate.

The most effective workplace tobacco control strategies have used comprehensive approaches, implementing tobacco bans as well as focusing on those at high risk (23).

SCREENING

Screening is the systematic application of a test to identify individuals at risk of a specific disease. The goal is for people who have not sought medical attention to benefit from further investigation or direct preventive action. Effectively implemented medical screening can prevent disability and death and improve quality of life. Screening tests are available for some chronic diseases, including cardiovascular disease, diabetes, and several site-specific cancers (24).

The disease or disorder to be considered for screening must be well defined, of public health importance and of known prevalence in the population. An effective, affordable and acceptable treatment must be available to all those who require it (25).

In general, the number of proven screening procedures is limited, although notable exceptions include the following:

» screening for elevated risk of cardiovascular disease using an overall risk approach;

» screening for early detection of breast and cervical cancer, in countries with sufficient resources to provide appropriate treatment.

SPOTLIGHT
WORKPLACE HEALTH IN THE UNITED STATES

Johnson & Johnson's Health & Wellness Program seeks to reduce behavioural and psychosocial risk factors, increase healthy behaviours, detect disease early, and manage chronic diseases. The programme provides preventive services as well as services during and after a major medical event.

After almost three years, improvement was seen in eight out of 13 risk categories for employees. Risk reductions were significant for tobacco use, aerobic exercise, high blood pressure, high cholesterol, dietary fibre intake, seat-belt use, and drinking and driving habits. The programme also resulted in financial benefits to Johnson & Johnson in the amount of money saved per employee per year on medical expenses. These savings increased substantially after the second year (26, 27).

SPOTLIGHT
CERVICAL CANCER SCREENING IN COSTA RICA

Cervical cancer remains a major health problem, particularly in low and middle income countries. Yet it can be prevented and cured if detected early. Effective screening programmes for cervical cancer in low and middle income countries can help reduce cervical cancer incidence and mortality. For example, in a number of Latin American countries, cervical cytology screening programmes have been in place for more than three decades and show some positive results.

In Costa Rica, cytology screening has been available to women aged 15 years and older since 1970. Some 250 000 smears are carried out every year, and more than 85% of eligible women have been screened at least once. However, nationwide coverage varies greatly and coverage of rural areas is still inadequate. Although the incidence of cervical cancer remained stable from 1983 to 1991, it declined significantly more recently, with a 3.6% decrease in annual incidence in 1993–1997 as compared with 1988–1992 (28).

CLINICAL PREVENTION

Clinical prevention is designed either to reduce the risk of disease onset or to reduce complications of disease in people living with disease. There are a number of highly effective clinical interventions that, when properly delivered, can reduce death and disease and improve the quality of life of people at risk of, or living with, chronic diseases. These include supporting behaviour change, the use of pharmacological agents and surgery. One example – combination drug therapy (aspirin, beta blocker, diuretic, statin) for people with an estimated overall risk of a cardiovascular event above 5% over the next 10 years – was shown to be very cost-effective in all regions by the WHO-CHOICE project.

SUCCESS FACTORS

A combination of interventions is required to realize the full potential of risk reduction.

» Treatment approaches based on overall risk, which take into account several risk factors at once, are more cost-effective than those based on arbitrary cut-off levels of individual risk factors.

» For some diseases (such as cataract) single, highly cost-effective interventions are available.

REDUCING THE RISKS OF DISEASE ONSET

Clinical interventions are a key component of comprehensive programmes for reducing the likelihood of disease onset. Individuals are at highest risk when they have several risk factors or when they have established disease. To reduce the likelihood of disease onset among high-risk individuals, screening and treatment need to be based on an assessment of overall risk (as determined by multiple rather than single risk factors).

A FOCUS ON OVERALL RISK

Overall risk refers to the probability of disease onset over a specified time period. Cut points for defining individuals at high risk and requiring clinical intervention need to be based on consideration of the desires of informed patients, the availability of cost-effective interventions and the risks and benefits of interventions, as well as their cost. Ideally, the assessment of future risk should be based on locally relevant data; unfortunately this is not usually available and risks are often assessed on the basis of data from other populations (*29*).

The overall risk of new cardiovascular disease events can be estimated by taking into account several risk factors. The charts on the following pages make it simple to calculate a person's risk. These charts estimate the risk of a cardiovascular event per 100 people over the next five years among people without previous symptomatic cardiovascular disease. They are used by identifying the category relating to a person's sex, diabetic status, tobacco-use history and age (*30*).

INTERVENTIONS FOR HIGH-RISK INDIVIDUALS

There are several highly effective clinical interventions appropriate for individuals at high risk. The benefits of the intervention must, however, clearly outweigh any danger, such as unwanted pharmacological effects. Interventions should be evidence-based, and they should also consider local needs and resource constraints. Sufficient resources must be available to provide the intervention to all those identified as in need.

REDUCING THE RISKS IN ESTABLISHED DISEASE

For cardiovascular disease and diabetes in particular, evidence-based approaches to reducing the risk of adverse outcomes in people with the disease are very similar to the approaches used to reduce disease onset. The major difference is that the likelihood of future clinical events is much greater once disease is established.

New Zealand cardiovascular risk charts
Risk level: women

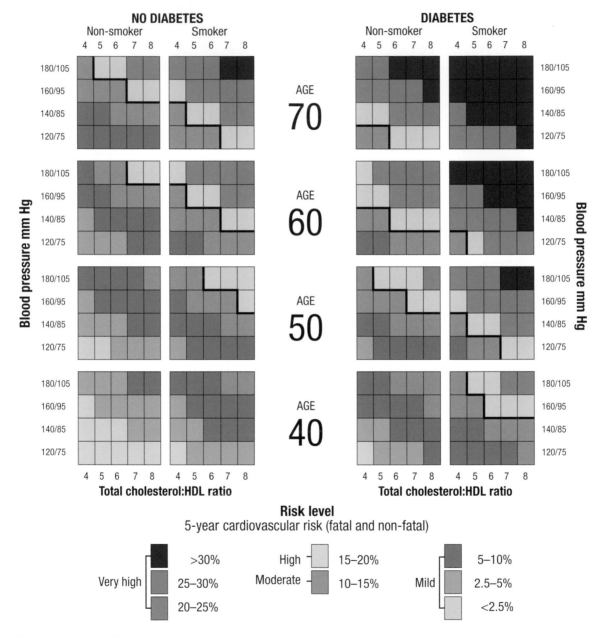

Risk level
5-year cardiovascular risk (fatal and non-fatal)

Very high	>30%	
	25–30%	
	20–25%	
High	15–20%	
Moderate	10–15%	
Mild	5–10%	
	2.5–5%	
	<2.5%	

How to use the charts
- Identify the chart relating to the person's sex, diabetic status, smoking history and age.
- Within the chart choose the cell nearest to the person's age, blood pressure and total cholesterol:HDL ratio. When the systolic and diastolic values fall in different risk levels, the higher category applies.
- For example, the lower left cell contains all non-smokers without diabetes who are less than 45 years old and have a total cholesterol:HDL ratio less than 4.5 and a blood pressure less than 130/80 mm Hg. People who fall exactly on a threshold between cells are placed in the cell indicating higher risk.

New Zealand cardiovascular risk charts
Risk level: men

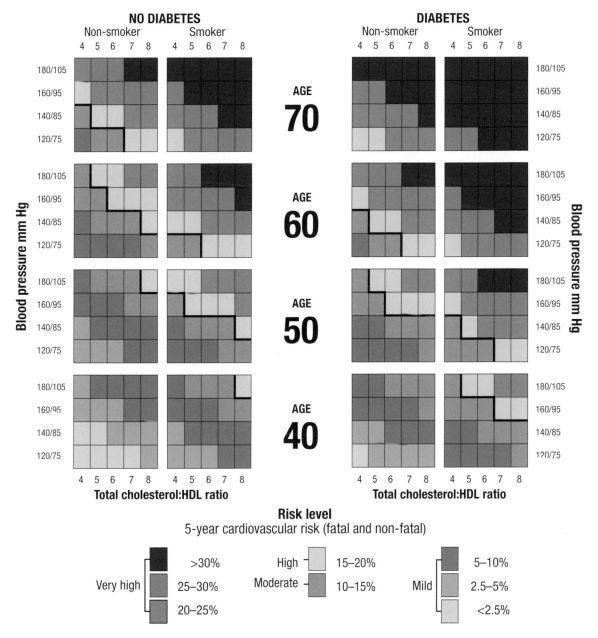

Risk level
5-year cardiovascular risk (fatal and non-fatal)

Very high	>30%	High	15–20%	5–10%
	25–30%	Moderate	10–15%	Mild 2.5–5%
	20–25%			<2.5%

How to use the charts
- Identify the chart relating to the person's sex, diabetic status, smoking history and age.
- Within the chart choose the cell nearest to the person's age, blood pressure and total cholesterol:HDL ratio. When the systolic and diastolic values fall in different risk levels, the higher category applies.
- For example, the lower left cell contains all non-smokers without diabetes who are less than 45 years old and have a total cholesterol:HDL ratio less than 4.5 and a blood pressure less than 130/80 mm Hg. People who fall exactly on a threshold between cells are placed in the cell indicating higher risk.

Highly effective interventions exist for reducing the risk of cardiovascular events in patients with diabetes and/or established cardiovascular disease. They include the following:

» Behavioural interventions: including those for tobacco cessation, increased physical activity and dietary change, with the promotion of weight loss if appropriate. Together, these may achieve a risk reduction of over 60% in people with established heart disease, and are also a key part of achieving good blood glucose control in people with diabetes (*31*).

» Pharmacological interventions: including aspirin, beta-blockers, angiotensin converting enzyme inhibitors and statins. A combination of all four of these is expected to reduce the risk of recurrent myocardial infarction by 75%.

People with established cardiovascular disease are at the highest risk of cardiovascular death and account for half of all cardiovascular deaths. For these people, international guidelines recommend long-term antiplatelet, blood pressure lowering and cholesterol lowering therapies. However, treatment gaps are substantial in all countries, in part because of the cost and complexity of multiple drug use.

POTENTIAL OF FIXED DOSE COMBINATION THERAPY

One strategy that has been proposed to reduce these barriers is a fixed dose combination pill (now commonly known as a *polypill*). Because each component apparently works in addition to the others, net benefits are anticipated to be substantial – risk reduction of more than two thirds within a few years of treatment – although more research is

SPOTLIGHT
TOBACCO CESSATION SERVICES IN THE UNITED KINGDOM

The United Kingdom's National Health Service (NHS) Stop Smoking Services were set up in 1999 in Health Action Zones, which were established in areas of deprivation and poor health in order to help tackle health inequalities. Following successful implementation in these areas, the services were made available across England to all smokers. Smokers set a date with the help of their adviser, and are then supported through the first stages of their attempt to stop smoking and followed-up after four weeks. A large increase in funding was made available and a demanding national target was set: 800 000 smokers to have stopped at the four-week follow-up stage by March 2006. It is planned that an electronic appointments system will be available to smokers to book appointments with the NHS Stop Smoking Services. This is supported by a tobacco control strategy including the media (in an education and information role), strengthening of regional and local action, reducing supply and availability, reducing tobacco promotion, and reducing exposure to second-hand smoke.

Results for the period April 2004–March 2005 show that around 300 000 smokers had successfully stopped at the four-week follow-up stage compared with about 205 000 the year before (an increase of 45%). Initial findings also show that equity of access to treatment is good, although success rates are lower among disadvantaged groups.

needed. Fixed dose combinations are now a core component of care for people with HIV/AIDS, tuberculosis and malaria. As well as improving clinical outcomes, they simplify distribution of multiple medications, which can be an important advantage in a resource-limited health-care setting.

The major challenge remains one of implementation – new strategies are required for the many millions of under-treated individuals with established cardiovascular disease in low and middle income countries. Ideally, these strategies should integrate with systems for other long-term medication delivery, such as those for HIV/AIDS, and complement population-wide measures to address the causes of cardiovascular disease.

The components of a polypill are no longer covered by patent restrictions and could be produced at a cost of little more than US$ 1 per patient per month. For people with cardiovascular disease in low and middle income countries, access to preventive care is usually dependent upon their ability to pay, and hence it is this large, underserved group that stands to gain most from a polypill (*32, 33*).

DISEASE MANAGEMENT

The previous sections of this chapter have shown that there are highly effective and cost-effective interventions to reduce the morbidity and mortality attributable to chronic diseases. Yet in many places, effective interventions for chronic diseases are poorly delivered or are not available at all.

Specific reasons for poor or absent delivery of chronic disease interventions vary between countries and between regions within countries. In some settings, lack of human, physical and financial resources are the major constraining factors. In other settings, resources are available but are used in a fragmented and inefficient manner. Factors to take into account include the following:

» evidence-based decision support tools can improve the delivery of effective care for chronic diseases;

» effective clinical information systems, including patient registries, are an essential tool for providing the continuity of care necessary for chronic diseases;

SPOTLIGHT
CHRONIC DISEASE MANAGEMENT IN SOUTH AFRICA

In a rural South African setting, a nurse-led chronic disease management programme for high blood pressure, diabetes, asthma, and epilepsy was established as part of primary health care for a population of around 200 000 people. The programme included the introduction of: clinic-held treatment cards and registries; diagnostic and management protocols; self-management support services; and regular, planned follow-up with a clinic nurse.

Nurses were able to improve disease control among most of the patients: 68% of patients with high blood pressure, 82% of those with diabetes, and 84% of those with asthma (*34*).

SPOTLIGHT

HEALTH-CARE QUALITY IMPROVEMENT IN THE RUSSIAN FEDERATION

Tula is an industrial town in the Russian Federation in which cardiovascular disease is a leading cause of death, accounting for 55% of adult mortality. High blood pressure prevalence is estimated at 27% and is considered to be a primary contributor to this mortality rate.

In 1998 the Central Public Health Research Institute of the Russian Ministry of Health and the Tula Oblast Health Authority, together with international partners, began an attempt to improve care for patients with high blood pressure. Five health-care facilities, each with a multidisciplinary team of staff, were involved in the decision-making and planning of the project. Goals included:

» developing evidence-based guidelines for high blood pressure care at the primary care level;

» changing the delivery of care for high blood pressure to reflect the new guidelines;

» promoting healthy behaviours to prevent the complications of high blood pressure;

» reallocation of financial and human resources to facilitate implementation of these services.

Positive outcomes included a sevenfold increase in the number of patients managed at primary care level. There was a 70% success rate in controlling high blood pressure, an 85% reduction in admissions for high blood pressure, and net savings for overall high blood pressure care costs of 23%. Other recent results from Russia, however, have not been so impressive (*35*).

The quality improvement project was expanded during Phase II (2000–2002) to all 289 general practitioner practices covering the whole population of the Tula region, and Phase III (national scale up) for integrated chronic disease prevention and control was launched in December 2002 (*36*).

» the provision of multidisciplinary health-care teams can be a highly effective approach to improving chronic disease care;

» the support of patient self-management is a core element of effective chronic disease care.

RELEVANCE FOR HIV/AIDS

These factors are also applicable to HIV/AIDS care. Health specialists are increasingly viewing HIV/AIDS as a chronic condition that requires comprehensive health services similar to those needed for heart disease and diabetes. Countries can obtain greater efficiency from their health systems by combining disease management for all chronic conditions.

USE OF PATIENT INFORMATION SYSTEMS

Well-designed, locally relevant and sustainable clinical information systems are essential if the goal of coordinated long-term care is to be achieved. They enable the organization of patient information, tracking and planning of patient care, provision of support for patient self-management, and scheduling of patient follow-up.

Clinical information systems are effective when they encourage communication between clinical team members and patients. They can take a variety of forms, and effective systems can be created even in very resource-poor settings. They may be paper-based, such as a chronic disease register kept in a notebook, and be linked to patient records, computerized, or a combination of the two.

MULTIDISCIPLINARY HEALTH-CARE TEAMS

One of the characteristics of most chronic diseases is that the care required for them cuts across several different health-care disciplines. Multidisciplinary health-care teams, centred on primary health care, are an effective means in all settings of achieving this goal and of improving health-care outcomes (37).

WORKING SUCCESSFULLY IN RESOURCE-POOR SETTINGS

The long list of health-care disciplines that ideally should be available for individuals with chronic diseases may appear to be unrealistic in resource-poor settings. It is possible, however, to provide some of the core skills from these disciplines in other ways (by training primary health-care workers in key elements of chronic disease management, for example). It may be possible to provide core aspects of effective health care that in more resourced settings would be provided by health professionals from several different disciplines.

USE OF EVIDENCE-BASED DECISION SUPPORT TOOLS

The development and implementation of evidence-based treatment guidelines is fundamental to putting evidence into practice. Guidelines have been defined as "systematically developed statements (recommendations) to assist practitioner and patient decisions about appropriate health care for specific clinical circumstances" (38). They draw on the best research evidence available at the time. The production of an evidence-based guideline is a resource-intensive and time consuming process. Nonetheless, evidence-based guidelines are available for many chronic diseases (see, for example, http://www.guideline.gov), and guidance on adapting them to specific national or local circumstances has been described. Of course, guidelines only work if they are used appropriately (39, 40).

SUCCESS FACTORS

The evidence suggests that the more specific and focused the approach to implementation, the more likely that practice will change in the direction recommended by a guideline. For example, simply providing information about the guideline is likely to have little impact, but linking the guideline to workshops or outreach training sessions and providing prompts within medical records are much more likely to change practice (41).

SPOTLIGHT
IMPROVING DIABETES CARE IN MEXICO

The Secretariat of Health of Mexico has launched a "crusade for the quality of health services" to provide better health care to people with chronic diseases. A one-year pilot project was conducted in the State of Veracruz, with in-service training of primary care personnel and the implementation of a structured diabetes education programme. Primary health-care teams were trained to adopt a quality improvement methodology. Among the innovations in primary health centres were the organization of diabetes clinics, collective medical visits for self-support groups of people with diabetes, and training people with diabetes to be community health workers.

The number of people with diabetes and good control increased from 28% to 39% in the intervention group, while among those receiving usual care the proportion only increased from 21% to 28%. Documented foot care education increased to 76% of patients in the intervention group and only to 34% elsewhere. The proportion of patients using insulin increased among the intervention group from 3.5% to 7.1%, while it remained at 0.9% among those receiving usual care (42).

SPOTLIGHT
CHRONIC DISEASE SELF-MANAGEMENT IN CHINA

A chronic disease self-management programme was developed in Shanghai from 1999 to 2001. The programme was conducted by trained volunteer lay leaders and included exercise, the use of cognitive symptom-management techniques, nutrition, fatigue and sleep management, use of medications, management of fear, anger, and depression, communication with health professionals, problem-solving and decision-making.

The programme significantly improved participants' health behaviour, confidence and health status, and reduced the number of hospitalizations after six months. The programme has been implemented in 13 communities and six districts of Shanghai, and is being replicated in other cities (*43*).

SPOTLIGHT
COMMUNITY-BASED REHABILITATION IN INDIA

In rural south India, permanently blind people were supported with community-based rehabilitation. This included mobility training and training to perform normal daily activities. Quality of life improved for some 95% of participants (*44*).

SPOTLIGHT
COMMUNITY-BASED REHABILITATION IN PAKISTAN

In Pakistan, volunteer local supervisors from targeted communities (villages and slum areas) were taught to identify and train people with disabilities. One to two years after training, 80% of participants showed improvement in function (*45*).

SUPPORT FOR PATIENT SELF-MANAGEMENT

Self-management for people with chronic disease is now widely recognized as a necessary part of treatment. Interventions that aim to improve the ability of patients and their carers to manage conditions can be highly effective and are an essential component of chronic disease care (*46*).

REHABILITATION

Chronic diseases are major causes of disability, including blindness, lower limb amputation, motor and sensory dysfunction following stroke, chronic pain, and impaired functioning following myocardial infarction.

Rehabilitation is intended to enable people to continue to live full lives as part of society. In some conditions, notably after myocardial infarction, rehabilitation reduces mortality. Multidisciplinary and intensive rehabilitation programmes, common in high income countries, are typically not feasible in low and middle income countries. However, community-based rehabilitation can provide effective rehabilitation in these countries.

EVIDENCE OF EFFECTIVENESS

» Rehabilitation services for patients following a stroke and living at home can improve independence (*47*).

» Multidisciplinary rehabilitation services in patients with chronic low back pain can reduce pain and improve function (*48*).

» Cardiac rehabilitation (following myocardial infarction), with a focus on exercise, is associated with a significant reduction in mortality (*49–51*).

PROVIDING REHABILITATION SERVICES IN DEVELOPING COUNTRIES

Rehabilitation services are usually provided by a team of specialized personnel, including medical doctors, dentists, prosthetists, physiotherapists, occupational therapists, social workers, psychologists, speech therapists, audiologists and mobility instructors. In many low and middle income countries, this rehabilitation approach is not feasible owing to shortages of health workers and other resource constraints.

In these situations, community-based rehabilitation is a viable alternative, using and building on the community's resources as well as those offered at district, provincial and central levels. Community-based rehabilitation is implemented through the combined efforts of people with disabilities, their families, organizations and communities, as well as the relevant governmental and nongovernmental health, education, vocational, social and other services. Such efforts are being made in more than 90 (mostly low and middle income) countries. The focus has expanded to health care, education, livelihood opportunities and participation/inclusion. As an overall approach, it has not been rigorously evaluated but site-specific evidence is generally positive.

PALLIATIVE CARE

Palliative care concentrates on the management of life-threatening chronic diseases and on supporting people so that they can achieve the best quality of life possible. Although typically associated with life-threatening cancer, it is often needed in other chronic conditions. Palliative care ranges from personal care and assistance in daily living to counselling and pain management. Palliative care is an urgent need worldwide. It is an integral part of long-term care, and even when there is no cure, can improve quality of life and provide a painless and peaceful end to life.

Approaches to providing palliative care will be influenced by health-care infrastructure and resources as well as local cultural and religious values. The current evidence provides little guidance on whether one approach is superior to another and suggests that further studies would be useful (52–54).

SPOTLIGHT
PALLIATIVE CARE IN INDIA

In India, even though palliative care is included in the national cancer control programme, it is mainly provided by nongovernmental organizations. There have been some important successes that might be applied nationally. For example, the Pain and Palliative Care Society in Kerala has developed a network of 33 palliative care clinics providing free care to those who need it, with an emphasis on home care. Trained community volunteers helped in providing care together with families who were trained to ensure the continuity of treatment (55).

SPOTLIGHT
PALLIATIVE CARE IN SUB-SAHARAN AFRICA

"A Community Health Approach to Palliative Care for HIV and Cancer Patients in Africa" is a joint project in which five countries – Botswana, Ethiopia, Uganda, United Republic of Tanzania and Zimbabwe – and the World Health Organization are working together. The main goal of this project is to improve the quality of life of HIV/AIDS and cancer patients in sub-Saharan Africa by developing comprehensive palliative care programmes with a community health approach.

Uganda is the first country in Africa in which pain relief and palliative care for cancer and HIV/AIDS is a priority in the national health plan. Supported by the work of local nongovernmental organizations, particularly Hospice Africa Uganda, the Ministry of Health has included pain relief and palliative care in the home care package, based on a needs assessment of patients and their caregivers. Services include essential drugs for pain and other symptom relief, food and family support. Palliative care has worked in Uganda because a national programme founded on a public health approach was established, based on the WHO National Cancer Control Guidelines (56–58).

ZAHIDA BIBI
"I WAITED

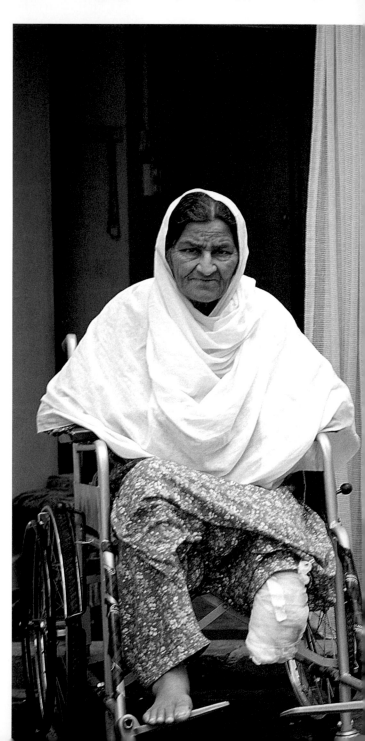

ZAHIDA BIBI HAS BEEN LIVING WITH DIABETES since the age of 45 and for several years was unaware that she had the disease. **"I was feeling tired and dizzy all the time. I was also having trouble remembering things and had to urinate a lot," she recalls. Zahida had consulted a doctor once, but was told that her blood test was normal.**

Name	Zahida Bibi
Age	65
Country	Pakistan
Diagnosis	Diabetes

After that, Zahida ignored her symptoms for eight long years before seeking medical care again, this time in Islamabad, 70 km from her home town. A second blood test finally established the nature of the problem and she started feeling much better almost immediately after taking her first shot of insulin.

"TOO LONG"

PAKISTAN

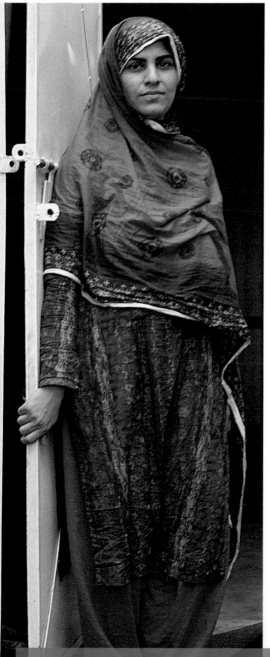

As is often true for people living with diabetes, Zahida recently developed serious complications which could have been avoided. One of her legs was amputated below the knee, as a result of an ulcer on her foot going untreated. "The doctor told me that it was connected with diabetes and that I waited too long and should have come to him at the first signs of infection," she says with regret.

Zahida holds her local hospital responsible for not having detected raised blood glucose in the first place, but admits that she should have reported the ulcer on her foot to her doctor much sooner. Now 65 years old, she is slowly recovering at home from the physical and emotional effects of surgery with the help of her son and daughter-in-law.

Many of the complications of diabetes, such as leg amputation, can be prevented with good health care.

CONCLUSION

Chronic diseases are already the major cause of death in almost all countries, and the threat to people's lives, their health and the economic development of their countries is growing fast. Yet, as this part of the report has shown, the knowledge exists to deal with this threat and to save millions of lives. Effective and cost-effective interventions, and the knowledge to implement them, have been shown to work in many countries.

If existing interventions are used together as part of a comprehensive, integrated approach, the global goal for preventing chronic diseases can be achieved. The only question is how governments, the private sector and civil society can work together to put such approaches into practice. If they do so in the ways outlined in the next part of the report, the global goal for chronic disease prevention and control will be achieved and millions of lives will be saved.

REFERENCES

1. Knowler WC, Barrett-Connor E, Fowler SE, Hamman RF, Lachin JM, Walker EA et al. Reduction in the incidence of type 2 diabetes with lifestyle intervention or metformin. *New England Journal of Medicine,* 2002, 346:393–403.

2. Pan XR, Li GW, Hu YH, Wang JX, Yang WY, An ZX et al. Effects of diet and exercise in preventing NIDDM in people with impaired glucose tolerance. The Da Qing IGT and Diabetes Study. *Diabetes Care*, 1997, 20:537–544.

3. Tuomilehto J, Lindstrom J, Eriksson JG, Valle TT, Hamalainen H, Ilanne-Parikka P et al. Prevention of type 2 diabetes mellitus by changes in lifestyle among subjects with impaired glucose tolerance. *New England Journal of Medicine,* 2001, 344:1343–1350.

4. Law MR, Wald NJ, Thompson SG. By how much and how quickly does reduction in serum cholesterol concentration lower risk of ischaemic heart disease? *BMJ*, 1994, 308:367–372.

5. Zatonski WA, Willett WC. *Dramatic decline in coronary heart disease mortality in Poland. Second look* (unpublished manuscript).

6. Zatonski WA, Willett W. Changes in dietary fat and declining coronary heart disease in Poland: population based study. *BMJ*, 2005, 331:187–188.

7. Vartiainen E, Jousilahti P, Alfthan G, Sundvall J, Pietinen P, Puska P. Cardiovascular risk factor changes in Finland, 1972–1997. *International Journal of Epidemiology*, 2000, 29:49–56.

8. Miguel-Baquilod M, Fishburn B, Santos J, Jones NR, Warren CW. Tobacco use among students aged 13–15 years – Philippines, 2000 and 2003. *Morbidity and Mortality Weekly Report*, 2005, 54:94–97.

9. Tan ASL, Arulanandam S, Chng CY, Vaithinathan R. Overview of legislation and tobacco control in Singapore. *International Journal of Tuberculosis and Lung Disease*, 2000, 4:1002–1008.

10. van Walbeek C. *Tobacco excise taxation in South Africa* (http://www.who.int/tobacco/training/success_stories/en/, accessed 5 July 2005).

11. Ewing R. Can the physical environment determine physical activity levels? *Exercise and Sports Science Reviews,* 2005, 33.

12. Handy S. *Critical assessment of the literature on the relationships among transportation, land use, and physical activity.* Paper prepared for the Transportation Research Board and the Institute of Medicine Committee on Physical Activity, Health, Transportation, and Land Use. Resource paper for *TRB Special Report 282*, January 2005.

13. *Built environment and the health of Bogotanos … a look at the neighborhood* [brochure]. Fundacion FES, Universidad de los Andes, Corporation de Universidades Centro de Bogota, Organizacion Panamericana de la Salud, US Centers for Disease Control and Prevention, International Union for Health and Physical Education.

14. Matsudo SM, Matsudo VR, Andrade DR, Araujo TL, Andrade E, de Oliveira L et al. Physical activity promotion: experiences and evaluation of the Agita Sao Paolo Program using the ecological mobile model. *Journal of Physical Activity and Health*, 2004, 1:81–97.

15. Nissinen A, Berrios X, Puska P. Community-based noncommunicable disease interventions: lessons from developed countries for developing ones. *Bulletin of the World Health Organization*, 2001, 79.963–970.

16. UNESCO/UNICEF/WHO/World Bank. *Focusing resources on effective school health: a FRESH start to enhancing the quality and equity of education. World Education Forum 2000, final report.* (http://portal.unesco.org/, accessed 6 July 2005).

17. Tian HG, Guo ZY, Hu G, Yu SJ, Sun W, Pietinen P et al. Changes in sodium intake and blood pressure in a community-based intervention project in China. *Journal of Human Hypertension*, 1995, 9:959–968.

18. Hoelscher DM, Feldman HA, Johnson CC, Lytle LA, Osganian SK, Parcel GS et al. School-based health education programs can be maintained over time: results from the CATCH Institutionalization Study. *Preventive Medicine,* 2004, 38:594–606.

19. Harvey J. *A feasibility study into healthier drinks vending in schools*. London, Food Standards Agency, Health Education Trust, 2004 (http://www.healthedtrust.com/pdf/%20FSA110304.pdf, accessed 5 July 2005).

20. Harvey J. *Vending healthy drinks. A guide for schools*. London, Food Standards Agency, Dairy Council, Health Education Trust, 2004 (http://www.healthedtrust.com/pdf/vendingmachinebooklet.pdf, accessed 5 July 2005).

21. *Dispensing junk: how school vending undermines efforts to feed children well*. Washington, DC, Center for Science in the Public Interest, 2004 (http://www.healthyschoolscampaign.org/news/downloads/dispensing_junk.pdf, accessed 5 July 2005).

22. Muto T, Yamauchi K. Evaluation of a multicomponent workplace health promotion program conducted in Japan for improving employees' cardiovascular disease risk factors. *Preventive Medicine,* 2001, 33:571–577.

23. Moher M, Hey K, Lancaster T. Workplace interventions for smoking cessation. *Cochrane Database of Systematic Reviews,* 2005, (2):CD003440.

24. Wald NJ. Guidance on terminology. *Journal of Medical Screening*, 2001, 8:56.

25. Strong K, Wald N, Miller A, Alwan A. Current concepts in screening for noncommunicable disease: World Health Organization Consultation Group Report on methodology of noncommunicable disease screening. *Journal of Medical Screening,* 2005, 12:12–19.

26. Goetzel RZ, Ozminkowski RJ, Bruno JA, Rutter KR, Isaac F, Wang S. The long-term impact of Johnson & Johnson's Health & Wellness Program on employee health risks. *Journal of Occupational and Environmental Medicine*, 2002, 44:417–424.

27. Ozminkowski RJ, Ling D, Goetzel RZ, Bruno JA, Rutter KR, Isaac F et al. Long-term impact of Johnson & Johnson's Health & Wellness Program on health care utilization and expenditures. *Journal of Occupational and Environmental Medicine*, 2002, 44:21–29.

28. Sankaranarayanan, R. Effective screening programmes for cervical cancer in low- and middle-income developing countries. *Bulletin of the World Health Organization*, 2002, 79:954–962.

29. Tang JL, Hu YH. Drugs for preventing cardiovascular disease in China. *BMJ*, 2005, 330:610–611.

30. *Assessing cardiovascular risk and treatment benefit.* Wellington, Ministry of Health, 2005 (http://www.nzgg.org.nz/guidelines/0035/CVD_Risk_Chart.pdf, accessed 5 July 2005).

31. *Prevention of recurrent heart attacks and strokes in low and middle income populations. Evidence-based recommendations for policy makers and health professionals.* Geneva, World Health Organization, 2003.

32. Wald N, Law M. A strategy to reduce cardiovascular disease by more than 80%. *BMJ*, 2003, 326:1419–1424.

33. Murray CJL, Lauer JA, Hutubessy RCW, Niessen L, Tomijima N, Rodgers A et al. Effectiveness and costs of interventions to lower systolic blood pressure and cholesterol: a global and regional analysis on reduction of cardiovascular-disease risk. *Lancet,* 2003, 361:717–725.

34. Coleman R, Gill G, Wilkinson D. Noncommunicable disease management in resource-poor settings: a primary care model from rural South Africa. *Bulletin of the World Health Organization,* 1998, 76:633–640.

35. Greenberg HM, Galyavitch AS, Ziganshina LE, Tinchurina MR, Chamidullin AG, Farmer RG. Hypertension management in a Russian polyclinic. *American Journal of Hypertension*, 2005, 18(Suppl. 1):A107.

36. Berwick DM. Lessons from developing nations on improving health care. *BMJ,* 2004, 328:1124–1129.

37. Sommer LS, Marton KI, Barbaccia JC, Randolph J. Physician, nurse and social worker collaboration in primary care for chronically ill seniors. *Archives of Internal Medicine,* 2000, 160:1825–1833.

38. Field MJ, Lohr KN, eds. *Guidelines for clinical practice – from development to use.* Washington, DC, National Academy Press, 1992.

39. *Guide for guidelines: a guide for clinical guideline development.* Brussels, International Diabetes Federation, 2003 (http://www.idf.org/home/index.cfm?node=1044, accessed 5 July 2005).

40. Grimshaw J, Eccles M, Tetroe J. Implementing clinical guidelines: current evidence and future implications. *Journal of Continuing Education in the Health Professions*, 2004, 24(Suppl. 1):S31–37.

41. Garg AX, Adhikari NK, McDonald H, Rosas-Arellano MP, Devereaux PJ, Beyene J et al. Effects of computerized clinical decision support systems on practitioner performance and patient outcomes: a systematic review. *JAMA*, 2005, 293:1223–1238.

42. *Proyecto Veracruz para el Mejoramiento de la Atención a la Diabetes (VIDA). Informe final [Veracruz Initiative for Diabetes Awareness (VIDA). Final report].* Washington, DC, Pan American Health Organization, 2005 (http://www.paho.org/common/Display.asp?Lang=S&RECID=7157, accessed 26 July 2005).

43. Fu D, Fu H, McGowan P, Shen YE, Zhu L, Yang H et al. Implementation and quantitative evaluation of chronic disease self-management programme in Shanghai, China: randomized controlled trial. *Bulletin of the World Health Organization*, 2003, 81:174–182.

44. Vijayakumar V, John RK, Datta D, Thulasiraj RD, Nirmalan PK. Quality of life after community-based rehabilitation for blind persons in a rural population of South India. *Indian Journal of Ophthalmology,* 2004, 52:331–335.

45. Finnstam J, Grimby G, Nelson G, Rashid S. Evaluation of community-based rehabilitation in Punjab, Pakistan: I: Use of the WHO manual, 'Training disabled people in the community'. *International Disability Studies*, 1988;10:54–58.

46. Bodenheimer T, Lorig K, Holman H, Grumbach K. Patient self-management of chronic disease in primary care. *JAMA*, 2002, 20:2469–2475.

47. Therapy-based rehabilitation services for stroke patients at home. *Cochrane Database of Systematic Reviews,* 2003, (1):CD002925.

48. Guzman J, Esmail R, Karjalainen K, Malmivaara A, Irvin E, Bombardier C. Multidisciplinary bio-psycho-social rehabilitation for chronic low-back pain. *Cochrane Database of Systematic Reviews*, 2002, (1):CD000963.

49. Jolliffe JA, Rees K, Taylor RS, Thompson D, Oldridge N, Ebrahim S. Exercise-based rehabilitation for coronary heart disease. *Cochrane Database of Systematic Reviews,* 2001, (1):CD001800.

50. Oldridge NB, Guyatt GH, Fischer ME, Rimm AA. Cardiac rehabilitation after myocardial infarction. Combined experience of randomized clinical trials. *JAMA*, 1988, 260:945–950.

51. Review: exercise-based cardiac rehabilitation reduces all-cause and cardiac mortality in coronary heart disease. *ACP Journal Club*, 2004, 141:62.

52. Salisbury C, Bosanquet N, Wilkinson EK, Franks PJ, Kite S, Lorentzon M et al. The impact of different models of specialist palliative care on patients' quality of life: a systematic literature review. *Palliative Medicine*, 1999, 13:3–17.

53. Wilkinson EK, Salisbury C, Bosanquet N, Franks PJ, Kite S, Lorentzon M et al. Patient and carer preference for, and satisfaction with, specialist models of palliative care: a systematic literature review. *Palliative Medicine*, 1999, 13:197–216.

54. Hearn J, Higginson IJ. Do specialist palliative care teams improve outcomes for cancer patients? A systematic literature review. *Palliative Medicine*, 1998, 12:317–332.

55. Bollini P, Venkateswaran C, Sureshkumar K. Palliative care in Kerala, India: a model for resource-poor settings. *Onkologie*, 2004, 27:138–142.

56. Stjernsward J. Uganda: initiating a government public health approach to pain relief and palliative care. *Journal of Pain and Symptom Management*, 2002, 24:257–264.

57. Sepulveda C, Habivambere V, Amandua J, Borok M, Kikule E, Mudanga B et al. Quality care at the end of life in Africa. *BMJ*, 2003, 327:209–213.

58. Spence D, Merriman A, Binagwaho A. Palliative care in Africa and the Caribbean. *PLoS Medicine*, 2004, 1:e5.

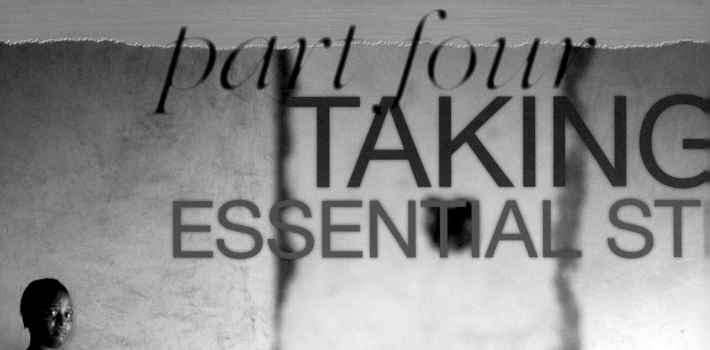

part four

TAKING

ESSENTIAL STE

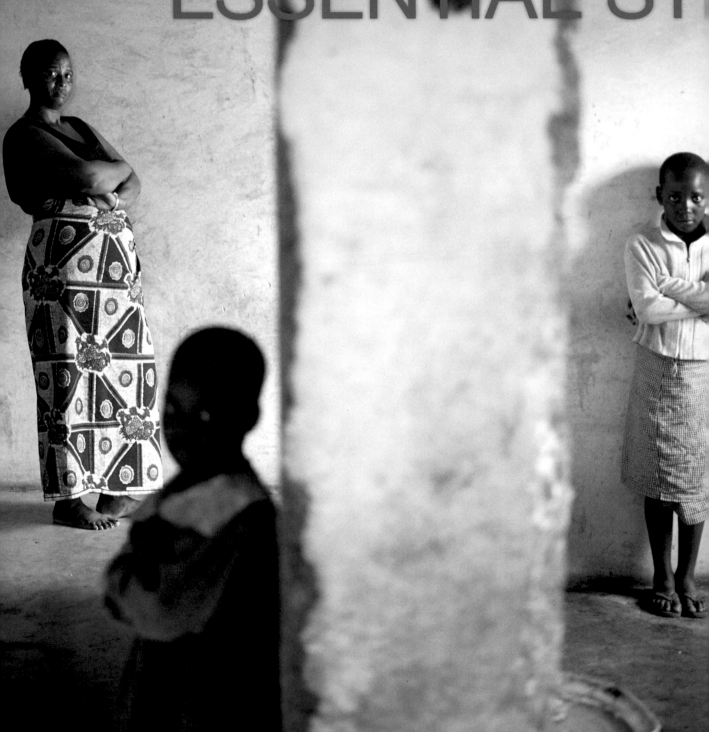

ACTION:
'S FOR SUCCESS

This part of the report outlines the steps that ministries of health can follow to implement successfully the interventions presented in Part Three. The opportunity exists to make a major contribution to the prevention and control of chronic diseases, and to achieve the global goal for chronic disease prevention and control by 2015.

Each country has its own set of health functions at national and sub-national levels. While there cannot be a single prescription for implementation, there are core policy functions that should be undertaken at the national level. A national unifying framework will ensure that actions at all levels are linked and mutually supportive. Other government departments, the private sector, civil society and international organizations all have crucial roles to play.

face to face
WITH **CHRONIC DISEASE**

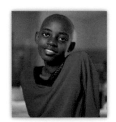

MARIAM JOHN
"I know I can make it"

144

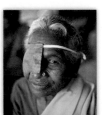

KUZHANTHIAMMAL
Waking up to vision

156

1 Providing a unifying framework – the role of government

A sound and explicit government policy is the key to effective prevention and control of chronic diseases. This chapter outlines a stepwise framework that ministries of health can use to create a policy and regulatory environment in which other sectors can operate successfully. The guidance and recommendations provided in this chapter may be used by national as well as sub-national level policy-makers and planners.

>> The national government's **unifying framework** for chronic disease prevention and control will ensure that actions at all levels and by all sectors are mutually supportive

>> **Integrated** prevention and control strategies are most effective – focusing on the common risk factors and cutting across specific diseases

>> **Comprehensive** public health action requires a combination of interventions for the whole population and for individuals

>> Most countries will not have the resources immediately to do everything that would ideally be done. Those activities which are most feasible given the existing context should be implemented first: this is the **stepwise** approach

>> Because major determinants of the chronic disease burden lie outside the health sector, **intersectoral** action is necessary at all stages of policy formulation and implementation

>> Locally relevant and explicit **milestones** should be established for each step and at each level of intervention, with a particular focus on reducing health inequalities

The stepwise framework

1 PLANNING STEP 1
Estimate population need and advocate for action

2 PLANNING STEP 2
Formulate and adopt policy

3 PLANNING STEP 3
Identify policy implementation steps

Policy implementation steps	Population-wide interventions		Interventions for individuals
	National level	Sub-national level	
Implementation step 1 **CORE**	Interventions that are feasible to implement with existing resources in the short term.		
Implementation step 2 **EXPANDED**	Interventions that are possible to implement with a realistically projected increase in, or reallocation of, resources in the medium term.		
Implementation step 3 **DESIRABLE**	Evidence-based interventions which are beyond the reach of existing resources.		

Introduction to the stepwis

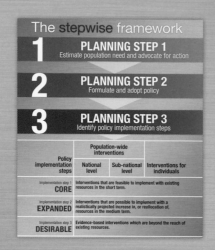

The stepwise framework offers a flexible and practical approach to assist ministries of health in balancing diverse needs and priorities while implementing evidence-based interventions.

ramework

OVERVIEW

The stepwise framework includes three main planning steps and three main implementation steps, which will be described in detail later in this chapter.

The first planning step is to assess the current risk factor profile of the population. This is followed by making the case for action.

The second planning step is to formulate and adopt chronic disease policy.

The third planning step is to identify the most effective means of implementing this policy. The chosen combination of interventions can be considered as levers for putting policy into practice with maximum effect.

Planning is followed by a series of implementation steps: core, expanded and desirable. The chosen combination of interventions for core implementation forms the starting point and the foundation for further action.

This chapter suggests specific milestones for different stages of implementation. These are not prescriptive, because each country must consider a range of factors in deciding the package of interventions that constitute the first, core implementation step, including the capacity for implementation, acceptability and political support.

THE REALITY OF PLANNING

While the stepwise framework has the benefits of offering a rational process and rallying multiple disciplines around an acceptable course of action, it does not automatically resolve the difficulties encountered in planning chronic disease prevention and control programmes. The reality is that public health action is incremental and opportunistic, reversing and changing directions constantly. The different planning and implementation steps might in fact overlap with one another depending on the unique situation.

The priority accorded to different health programmes is partly a result of the broader political climate. It is important to identify, and ideally predict, the national or sub-national political climate and to capitalize on opportunities.

The priorities of individual political leaders can be dramatically shaped by private experiences. There are many examples of leaders who, after being personally touched by disease, have subsequently made that disease a new national priority for action. These people can be important allies for change.

1 PLANNIN
Estimate population nee

Although some disease burden information may be available, the distribution of risk factors among the population is the key information required by countries in their planning of prevention and control programmes. This information predicts the future burden of disease; it must then be synthesized and disseminated in a way that successfully argues the case for the adoption of relevant policies.

ESTIMATING NEED

WHO has developed a tool to help low and middle income countries assess their risk factor profiles – the STEPwise approach to Surveillance (STEPS).

WHO STEPS focuses on building capacity in low and middle income countries to collect small amounts of high-quality risk factor data:

» Step 1: collect questionnaire-based information about diet and physical activity, tobacco use and alcohol consumption;

» Step 2: use standardized physical measurements to collect data on blood pressure, height and weight;

» Step 3: expand physical measurements with the collection of blood samples for measurement of lipids and glucose status.

Although most countries have the resources for collecting data in the first two stages, the third is resource-intensive and not suited for all settings or sites. STEPS is designed to allow flexibility for local adaptation, and also offers expanded modules (such as oral health and stroke) while encouraging collection of standardized data (1).

STEP 1
nd advocate for action

SPOTLIGHT
ADVOCATING FOR ACTION
IN LATIN AMERICA AND
THE CARIBBEAN

he WHO Regional Office for the Americas (AMRO) held
series of workshops in collaboration with the Inter-
ational Union Against Cancer to advocate for cervical
ancer prevention policies and programmes in Latin
merica and the Caribbean. More than 300 key stake-
olders from ministries of health, nongovernmental
rganizations, medical and professional associations,
nd international agencies participated.

The workshops were structured to help build alliances
etween national governments and other stakeholders
nd to create a forum for the exchange of technical
formation. The objectives were to achieve consensus
n the need for, and the process by which, cervical
ancer prevention and control could be placed on the
genda, and to encourage countries to strengthen or
evelop their cervical cancer prevention and control
rogrammes.

Following the workshops, more than 10 countries in
he region critically assessed their programmes with
ssistance from AMRO, devised strategic programme
lans and received seed funding to implement new
trategies for cervical cancer prevention. Through
eetings with ministers of health, joint planning and
echnical cooperation agendas have been established,
nd in the Caribbean Caucus of Ministers of Health a
trategic plan was presented and adopted for a sub-
egional approach to screening and treatment.

ADVOCATING FOR ACTION

Information on population need must be synthesized
and disseminated in a way that encourages policy
action at national level. Policy-makers should be
informed of national trends in risk factors, the current and projected problem of chronic diseases in the
country, and the existence of cost-effective interventions for prevention and control.

Communication methods for influencing policy-
makers include:

» media features, which influence the views of the
  general public (including, where relevant, voters)
  as well as policy-makers directly;

» identification and engagement of community
  leaders and other influential members of society
  who can spread the message in different forums;

» one-on-one meetings with policy-makers.

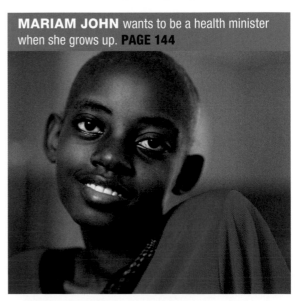

MARIAM JOHN wants to be a health minister
when she grows up. **PAGE 144**

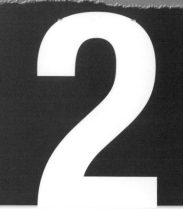

2 PLANNINC
Formulate ar

INDONESIA'S NATIONAL POLICY DEVELOPMENT

For many years the scale of the chronic disease problem in Indonesia had been concealed by a lack of reliable information. Prevention and control activities were scattered, fragmented and lacked coordination. Periodic household surveys later revealed that the proportion of deaths from chronic diseases doubled between 1980 and 2001 (from 25% to 49%). The economic implications and the pressing need to establish an integrated prevention platform at national, district and community levels became clear.

In 2001, inspired by the WHO Global Strategy on the Prevention and Control of Noncommunicable Diseases, Indonesia's Ministry of Health initiated a broad consultative process that resulted in a national consensus on chronic disease policy and strategy. A collaborative network for chronic disease surveillance, prevention and control was established, involving health programmes, professional organizations, nongovernmental organizations, educational institutions and other partners from both the public and private sectors (including those not directly concerned with health). The WHO STEPS manual was translated into Indonesian and implemented as part of the overall surveillance approach.

A national policy and strategy document was published by the Ministry of Health in 2004. The document recommends targeting major diseases that share common risk factors through surveillance, health promotion, prevention and reform of health services. The need for integrated, efficient and sustainable surveillance, prevention and control efforts has been recognized as a vital component of the national health development agenda.

The second planning step, after estimating population need and advocating for action, is to formulate and adopt policy. A policy sets out the vision for prevention and control of the major chronic diseases and provides the basis for action in the next 5–10 years. It is accompanied by plans and programmes that provide the means for implementing the policy.

The main goals of a public health policy for chronic disease prevention and control are similar to those of any health policy:

» improve the health of the population, especially the most disadvantaged;
» respond to needs and expectations of people who have chronic diseases;
» provide financial protection against the costs of ill-health.

In all countries, a **national** policy and planning framework is essential to give chronic diseases appropriate priority and to organize resources efficiently.

At the **sub-national level**, complementary policies, plans and programmes can be developed at the state, province, district, and/or municipal levels to respond to local circumstances.

GUIDING PRINCIPLES
Chronic disease policy should be based on the following guiding principles:
» comprehensive and integrated public health action;
» intersectoral action;
» a life course perspective;
» stepwise implementation based on local considerations and needs.

STEP 2
dopt policy

SPOTLIGHT
CHINA'S NATIONAL STRATEGY FOR CHRONIC DISEASE CONTROL

China's Ministry of Health, with the support of WHO and the cooperation of relevant sectors, has been developing a national plan for chronic disease prevention and control, which focuses on cardiovascular diseases, cancer, chronic obstructive pulmonary disease and diabetes. It is expected to be applicable to both the medium and long term, and include an action plan for 3–5 years. This follows an earlier programme of Cancer Prevention and Control in China (2004–2010) developed by the Ministry of Health.

The national plan aims to reduce the overall level of risk factors, to improve early detection and treatment and to provide accessible and affordable health services. It includes the development of national system of prevention and control, which will require comprehensive financing, multisectoral cooperation and the establishment of expert committees at the national and local levels. It will also involve capacity building and the establishment of a national surveillance system, as well as periodic surveys of nutrition and health (2).

COMPREHENSIVE AND INTEGRATED PUBLIC HEALTH ACTION

Comprehensive and integrated policies and plans are vital, because they minimize overlap and fragmentation in the health system. They should therefore:

» cut across specific diseases and focus on the common risk factors;
» encompass promotion, prevention, and control strategies;
» emphasize the management of the entire population over the management of specific subgroups;
» integrate across settings, such as health centres, schools, workplaces and communities;
» make explicit links to other government programmes and community-based organizations.

Programme implementation itself should also be comprehensive and integrated because:

» it is both impossible and unnecessary to have specific programmes for different chronic diseases;
» without a national organizing framework, there is a risk that initiatives may be developed or implemented independently of each other, and opportunities for synergies may not be realized.

INTERSECTORAL ACTION

Intersectoral action is necessary because, as reviewed in Part Two of this report, the underlying determinants of the chronic disease burden lie outside the health sector. These include poverty, lack of education and unhealthy environmental conditions. More proximal chronic disease risks, such as unhealthy diets and physical inactivity, are also influenced by sectors outside health, such as transport, agriculture and trade.

An intersectoral committee should be created for policy-making. At the national level, it should be convened by the ministry of health, but with representation from other relevant ministries and organizations.

Different sectors may have different and sometimes even conflicting priorities. In such situations, the health sector needs the capacity to provide leadership, to provide arguments for a win-win situation and to adapt to the agendas and priorities of other sectors.

PLANNING STEP 2
Formulate and adopt policy

SPOTLIGHT
A CHANGING NATIONAL HEALTH SYSTEM IN CHILE

In 2000, a national survey on living conditions and health, coupled with mortality data, clearly showed the large health inequalities and increasing magnitude of chronic diseases in Chile. Based on this information, the Government of Chile made a commitment to improving the health of the population and to improving health among the most disadvantaged groups. This led to the establishment of health objectives for 2010. Targets for chronic diseases include decreasing tobacco use, decreasing the prevalence of obesity in children and pregnant women, reducing physical inactivity and lowering mortality from cardiovascular diseases, cancers and respiratory diseases. Further targets include reducing the disability associated with diabetes, increasing oral health coverage, and increasing coverage of palliative care for people dying at home.

For 56 health conditions, 39 of which relate to chronic diseases, the Government committed itself to universal access to care, opportunity of care, quality of care, and financial coverage. Under this plan, private insurers must comply with the same regulations and guidelines as the public system.

Full participation of all stakeholders and of society at large under the stewardship of the Ministry of Health was crucial. Once the needs of the population were estimated, priorities were able to be set, thereby ensuring adequate distribution of resources.

LIFE COURSE PERSPECTIVE

Risk factors accumulate from fetal life through to adulthood. Because risk behaviours are commonly established in childhood and adolescence, prevention strategies should include school health programmes focused on promoting healthy diets, physical activity, and tobacco abstinence. Adolescents who have already adopted risk behaviours such as tobacco use, or who have intermediate risks such as obesity, should be targeted for specialized interventions. Population-wide approaches such as smoke-free environments, advertising bans and taxation of tobacco are also essential to protect child and adolescent health.

Rapid population ageing is another factor to be taken into consideration in policy development. The challenge for health policy-makers is to delay the onset of chronic diseases, and to improve functioning and quality of life.

STEPWISE IMPLEMENTATION

Most countries will not have the resources immediately to do everything implied by the overall policy. Core interventions that are feasible to implement within existing resources in the short term should be chosen first. Other activities are included in the "expanded" and "desirable" steps of implementation.

SPOTLIGHT
TONGA'S INTERSECTORAL POLICY DEVELOPMENT

During the 1980s and 1990s, Tonga became increasingly aware of the rising number of people with cardiovascular diseases, diabetes and complications of diabetes such as gangrene, kidney failure and blindness. The prevalence of diabetes in the adult population doubled to over 15% in 25 years, although the majority remained undiagnosed and untreated.

In 2003 clinicians, concerned public health staff and representatives of overseas development agencies met and conceived a national chronic disease strategy. Extensive consultations with stakeholders were held, and a survey was conducted to identify ongoing interventions.

The Government, churches, nongovernmental organizations and development agencies participated in a follow-up workshop. They produced the National Strategy to Prevent and Control Noncommunicable Diseases, based on the stepwise approach. A multisectoral committee was formed to coordinate the implementation of the strategy and advise the government, and four sub-committees on Physical Activity, Healthy Eating, Tobacco Control and Alcohol Misuse took responsibility for operational planning and implementation. The strategy was officially launched with national media coverage in March 2004 and later endorsed by cabinet.

Important achievements include:
- completion of a national survey on chronic diseases and risk factors, revision of the tobacco control act;
- development of a complete proposal to parliament for the establishment of a Health Promotion Unit funded by tobacco tax;
- inclusion of chronic disease control in the Millennium Development Goals for Tonga.

The strategy document has proved to be important in channelling external support and focusing resources on key interventions (3).

SUCCESS FACTORS
The following factors have been associated with success in policy formulation and adoption:

» a high-level political mandate to develop a national policy framework;

» a committed group of advocates who may be involved with estimating need, advocating for action, and developing the national policy and plan;

» international collaboration providing political and technical support;

» wide consultation in the process of drafting, consulting, reviewing and redrafting the policy until endorsement is achieved;

» an awareness that the process of consultation is as important as the content in generating support and ownership;

» development and implementation of a consistent communication strategy for all stages of the process;

» clarity of vision on a small set of outcome-oriented objectives.

3 PLANNING
Identify poli

The third planning step is to identify the best means by which policy can be implemented. The comprehensive approach requires a range of interventions to be implemented in a stepwise manner, depending on their feasibility and likely impact in the local conditions and taking into account potential constraints and barriers to action. Some of the selected interventions are primarily under the control of the health ministry, for example realigning health systems for chronic disease prevention and control. Others are primarily the responsibility of other government sectors or the legislative branch. In these cases, the ministry of health, as the primary steward of population health, should ensure coordination in cooperation with government partners.

A key decision – whether at global, regional, national or local level – is on how, where and when to proceed with different steps of implementation. This requires a blend of evidence, experience, judgement and advocacy. The most feasible activities should be selected first. Selecting a smaller number of activities and doing them well is likely to have more impact than tackling a large number and doing them haphazardly. Countries should also try to ensure that any new activities are complementary with those already under way locally, at state or province level, and nationally.

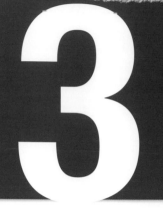

HEALTH POLICY LEVERS

Health financing

Legislation and regulation

Improving the built environment

Advocacy initiatives

Community mobilization

Health services organization and delivery

STEP 3
Implementation steps

HEALTH FINANCING

Health financing is an important mechanism by which policies and plans are translated into reality. Financing decisions based on principles of equity and effectiveness ensure adequate health-care access and coverage for all. Various financing components (funding, resource allocation, contracting and reimbursement) should be used to encourage the implementation of chronic disease prevention and control policies and plans.

Implementation step	Suggested milestones
STEP 1 CORE	» A line item for chronic disease prevention and control is included in the annual health budget.
STEP 2 EXPANDED	» Tobacco taxes are implemented and revenue is earmarked for population-wide interventions to reduce risk and promote health.
STEP 3 DESIRABLE	» The health financing system is reviewed and harmonized across diseases and levels of care, and designed to maximize equity and effectiveness. » The health benefit package includes preventive treatments and long-term care for chronic diseases.

As a first step, it is important that a line item for chronic disease prevention and control is included in the annual health budget. This will ensure that these activities are not lost among competing priorities.

PLANNING STEP 3
Identify policy implementation steps

SPOTLIGHT
THAIHEALTH

The Thai Health Promotion Foundation (ThaiHealth) was established in 2001 as a statutory, independent public organization, following the success of Thailand's nationwide anti-smoking movement. Funding of approximately US$ 50 million per year comes from a 2% excise tax on alcohol and cigarettes. Through policy advocacy and efforts by civil society groups, and with support from a series of studies managed by the Health System Research Institute, the Government and the Ministry of Finance became convinced that a Health Promotion Fund would be beneficial to the country. Its goal is to support activities that reduce risk factors and promote healthy behaviour.

ThaiHealth plays a catalytic and facilitating role, and focuses its support on activities that yield sustainable results. The organization has fostered health promotion alliances and networks and expanded its activities to reach as many people as possible. The "open grants" programme allows community-based and other organizations to secure funding for their heath promotion activities, and proactive grants support projects according to specific objectives such as model health-promoting schools. ThaiHealth has played a leading role in the movement against tobacco use, the campaigns to prevent drink-driving and reduce alcohol consumption, and activities to promote physical activity.

As reviewed in Part Three, an effective policy instrument for reducing the use of tobacco products is to tax them. Taxation also influences the consumption of food and drinks. Revenue from dedicated taxes can be earmarked for specific purposes. These taxes do not necessarily become part of consolidated revenue but can be allocated directly to a specific purpose such as population-wide prevention interventions.

A number of country and state governments have dedicated part of their tax revenues for particular health promotion initiatives. One innovative model to administer these tax revenues is the health promotion foundation (see spotlight, left).

The benefit package for chronic diseases should allow for preventive interventions as well as covering appropriate management of acute symptoms and long-term care (including rehabilitation and palliative and hospice care).

Financing long-term care is a major and growing challenge, as it is a major cost to health systems. Some countries use special premiums and general taxation funding, alone or in combination. Home-based care should also be included in financing schemes.

LEGISLATION AND REGULATION

As reviewed in Part Three, legislation and regulation are fundamental elements of effective public health policy and practice.

Implementation step		Suggested milestones
STEP 1	**CORE**	» Tobacco control legislation consistent with the WHO Framework Convention on Tobacco Control is enacted and enforced.
STEP 2	**EXPANDED**	» Food standards and food labelling legislation are enacted. » Action is taken to limit and control food marketing and advertising to children, to discourage availability of high fat, high salt and high sugar foods for children, and to promote eating of fruit and vegetables.
STEP 3	**DESIRABLE**	» Legislation is enacted to protect the rights of people with chronic disease and disability.

Specific legislative and regulatory policies that enhance prevention and control of chronic diseases include measures that:

» ban tobacco smoke in all indoor places;
» enforce bans on sales of tobacco products to youth;
» incorporate mandatory health warning labels on tobacco products;
» enforce tobacco advertising bans (including sponsoring of sports and cultural events);
» mandate appropriate labelling for foods sold in the domestic market, including warning statements, nutrient claims and nutrition information profiles;
» ensure that people with chronic disease and disabilities are accorded full human rights.

135

PLANNING STEP 3
Identify policy implementation steps

IMPROVING THE BUILT ENVIRONMENT

As reviewed in Part Three, built environment interventions have considerable potential to increase physical activity patterns. Urban design can positively influence walking, cycling and other forms of active transport.

Implementation step		Suggested milestones
STEP 1	**CORE**	» Leaders and decision-makers in urban design and transport sectors are informed of the impact that design and transport can have on physical activity patterns and chronic diseases.
STEP 2	**EXPANDED**	» Built environment and transport planning, design and construction decisions incorporate physical activity components.
STEP 3	**DESIRABLE**	» Future urban planning, transport design and construction of new buildings are conducive to active transport and physical activity.

SPOTLIGHT
IMPROVING THE BUILT ENVIRONMENT IN INDIA

In Chennai, India, the prevalence of diabetes is particularly high among middle income residents and people who undertake little physical activity. Realizing the importance of physical activity, residents mobilized resources from philanthropists and collected donations from residents to construct a park. A piece of land was identified and the local municipality was approached for building permission. The construction of the park was completed in 2002, with bushes, trees, fountains and a play area for children. The residents contribute a nominal annual fee for maintenance of the park.

A follow-up survey showed that there was a threefold increase in people undertaking regular physical activity (from less than 15% to 45%). Based on this success story, which was extensively reported in the local newspapers, another community in Chennai has also built a park (4).

Specific built environment interventions, such as the following, have considerable potential to increase physical activity patterns:

» provision of easily accessible, well-lit stairs in multi-story buildings;

» provision of cycle and walking paths in urban and rural communities;

» provision of accessible sports, fitness and recreation facilities;

» increased compact urban design rather than urban sprawl.

ADVOCACY INITIATIVES

As reviewed in Part Three, advocacy initiatives can support the initiation of national policies for chronic disease prevention. Advocacy includes a range of strategies for communicating risk, increasing motivation to change, and disseminating ideas through communities and societies.

Implementation step		Suggested milestones
STEP 1	CORE	» Opinion leaders are identified and engaged systematically to inform others about the growing burden of chronic diseases, the existence of effective interventions, and the comprehensive response that is needed.
STEP 2	EXPANDED	» Advocacy initiatives are strengthened to promote risk factor reduction among target populations.
STEP 3	DESIRABLE	» Comprehensive and integrated advocacy initiatives are implemented and incorporate multiple communication methods.

SPOTLIGHT
PROMOTING FRUIT AND VEGETABLE INTAKE IN ENGLAND

Current average consumption of fruit and vegetables in the United Kingdom is around three portions per day. The 5 A DAY Programme aims to increase this to the recommended daily level of around five portions, thereby contributing to the achievement of national targets on reducing mortality rates from cardiovascular disease and cancer, halting the year-on-year rise in obesity among children, and reducing inequalities in life expectancy.

The programme consists of several areas of work underpinned by an evaluation and monitoring programme. The 5 A DAY communications programme provides information and advice for consumers through television and radio advertising, leaflets, posters, booklets, a web site and magazine adverts and articles, and a 5 A DAY logo has been developed. Local and national partners include industry, government departments and other agencies. The School Fruit and Vegetable Scheme has led to nearly 2 million children aged four to six years receiving a free piece of fruit or vegetable each school day. A survey in October 2003 found that over a quarter of children and their families reported that they were eating more fruit at home after joining the scheme, including in lower socioeconomic groups. Research from December 2004 indicated that 37% of people claimed to have eaten "a lot more" or "a little more" fruit and vegetables over the previous 12 months. There was a year-on-year increase in awareness of the 5 A DAY message from 43% in October 2000 to 58% in October 2004.

137

PLANNING STEP 3
Identify policy implementation steps

COMMUNITY MOBILIZATION

Community mobilization, as illustrated in Part Three, is fundamental to creating and implementing successful and sustainable chronic disease prevention and control policies and programmes.

Implementation step		Suggested milestones
STEP 1	**CORE**	» Networks of community members and organizations, health professionals and policy-makers are established for information sharing, consultation and collaboration.
STEP 2	**EXPANDED**	» Community-based programmes for chronic disease prevention are formed, and then implemented and evaluated. » School health programmes for chronic disease prevention are systematically implemented.
STEP 3	**DESIRABLE**	» Communities assume responsibility for ongoing implementation and monitoring of chronic disease prevention programmes. » Employers implement chronic disease prevention and self-management activities in the workplace.

USING SCHOOLS TO PROMOTE HEALTHY DIETS AND PHYSICAL ACTIVITY

Large-scale school-based projects are being implemented in developing countries to reduce obesity, improve nutrition and increase physical activity. Brazil has recently required that 70% of the food offered through its national school meals programme should be minimally processed. Chile has included more fruits and vegetables in the national school meals programme. The Ministries of Health and Education in China have been fostering the health-promoting school concept (see spotlight, opposite). Malaysia, Mexico, the Republic of Korea, South Africa and Thailand have initiated similar programmes. In the Republic of Korea a healthy traditional diet was preserved through the joint efforts of dietitians and the government. The most promising programmes use culturally appropriate methods and messages (5).

SPOTLIGHT
SCHOOL-BASED PROJECTS IN CHINA

Since 1995, the Ministry of Health and the Ministry of Education in China have been collaborating with other domestic agencies and WHO to foster the concept of the "health-promoting school" as a means of improving health.

In Zhejiang Province, unhealthy diet is a major cause of both undernutrition and obesity among school-age children. In 2000, a health-promoting school project to improve nutrition was launched by the Provincial Education Commission and the Health Education Institute of the Centers for Disease Control and Prevention. The education sector was responsible for the management of schools, including improvements to the school environment as well as to the school health education curriculum. The health sector was responsible for issuing and supervising public health guidelines, monitoring the prevalence of disease, and prevention measures.

Zhejiang Province's health-promoting school project improved nutrition among 7500 students and their families and 800 teachers and school staff personnel. It actively engaged the target groups in planning, implementing and evaluating the interventions. Survey results revealed improvements in nutrition knowledge, attitudes and behaviour among all target groups (*6, 7*).

WORKPLACES

Workplaces provide unique points of access for interventions to reduce chronic disease risk factors and promote effective management of chronic conditions. A detailed analysis of workplace roles and functions is presented in the following chapter, in the section addressing the private sector.

139

PLANNING STEP 3
Identify policy implementation steps

HEALTH SERVICES ORGANIZATION AND DELIVERY

As Part Three demonstrated, reorientation of health services away from the traditional focus on acute health care, as well as a shift in budget allocation, are needed in many countries to respond adequately to chronic disease prevention and control.

PROMOTE THE USE OF EVIDENCE-BASED GUIDELINES

The introduction of integrated, evidence-based guidelines is one important method for promoting evidence-based care. Treatment guidelines should be approved at the national level, endorsed by local professional societies, and tailored to fit local contexts and resource constraints. Guidelines should be incorporated into assessment tools, patient registries and flowsheets in order to increase the likelihood of their use.

Implementation step	Suggested milestones
STEP 1 CORE	» A standard set of integrated clinical management guidelines is drafted and adopted at national level for implementation.
STEP 2 EXPANDED	» Clinical guidelines are integrated into everyday tools, for example visual prompts and chart reminders to help health-care workers provide evidence-based care.
STEP 3 DESIRABLE	» Ongoing monitoring and feedback regarding the implementation of clinical guidelines is provided at national, local, health centre and individual health-care provider levels.

EMPHASIZE PREVENTION AND MANAGEMENT BASED ON OVERALL RISK

As reviewed in Part Three, disease onset can be prevented through the identification and reduction of elevated risk, and complications of established disease can also be addressed using prevention strategies.

Risk prediction derived from multiple risk factors is more accurate than making treatment decisions on the basis of single risk factors. In most cases, a combination of interventions is required to realize the full potential of risk reduction.

Access to essential drugs should be a key component of the policy framework, focusing on rational selection, affordable prices and sustainable financing. For effective implementation of these drug policies, supply management systems need to be integrated into health system organization.

Implementation step	Suggested milestones
STEP 1 CORE	» Tobacco use is routinely assessed and tobacco cessation services are provided. » Affordable first-line chronic disease medications such as aspirin, as well as blood pressure and cholesterol-lowering drugs, are made available in primary health care.
STEP 2 EXPANDED	» Patients' levels of overall risk are systematically assessed and monitored during health-care visits. » Treatment interventions are based on locally tailored guidelines and on overall risk, rather than arbitrary cut-off levels of individual risk factors. » Second-line and third-line medications for chronic disease are made available and affordable.
STEP 3 DESIRABLE	» Comprehensive prevention programmes are available in primary health care.

PLANNING STEP 3
Identify policy implementation steps

ESTABLISH EFFECTIVE CLINICAL INFORMATION SYSTEMS

Clinical information systems assist in coordinating the overall operation of the health-care centre, organizing patient information, tracking and planning patient care and facilitating patient self-monitoring, as well as prompting health-care providers to schedule patient follow-up. Effective systems can be created regardless of resource level; they range from computerized registries to pencil-and-paper schemes, and they can be written or pictorial.

Implementation step	Suggested milestones
STEP 1　CORE	» Basic paper-based patient registries and medical records for patients with chronic disease are introduced into primary health care.
STEP 2　EXPANDED	» Computer-based patient registries and medical records for chronic disease patients are introduced into primary health care. » Patient information is shared between primary health care and specialty/hospital care.
STEP 3　DESIRABLE	» Health-care settings are electronically linked via a common clinical information system.

STRENGTHEN PATIENT SELF-MANAGEMENT

Patients need to be equipped with the tools and skills required to cope effectively with their conditions on a daily basis. A range of health-care workers and lay people can successfully teach these skills to individuals or groups, by telephone or electronically (see spotlight, below).

Implementation step	Suggested milestones
STEP 1 CORE	» Basic information about risk factors and (as appropriate), chronic diseases, is provided to patients. » Patients with chronic disease are informed about their role in self-managing, and about community-based resources.
STEP 2 EXPANDED	» Educational and skill-building workshops/group appointments on chronic disease management are provided to patients.
STEP 3 DESIRABLE	» Computerized patient self-assessment is used to generate individualized self-management plans. » Patients with chronic diseases are provided with supplementary self-management support by telephone or through the Internet.

SPOTLIGHT
A PATIENT-CENTRED APPROACH IN ENGLAND AND WALES

More than 17 million people in England and Wales have a chronic disease, which has a considerable impact on the National Health Service (NHS) and social care services. People with chronic health problems are more likely to see their general physician, be admitted as inpatients, and stay in hospital longer than those without these conditions.

The NHS Improvement Plan set out the government's strategy to improve care for people with chronic diseases, by moving away from reactive care based in acute systems, to a systematic, patient-centred approach. The national Public Service Agreement target focuses on improving health outcomes for people with chronic diseases by offering a personalized care plan for people most at risk, and reducing emergency bed days by 5% by 2008 through improved care in primary and community settings.

For the majority of people with chronic diseases, significant benefits follow when they receive increased support for managing their own symptoms and medication. To this end an Expert Patient Programme has been developed in the NHS. The programme has already involved many Primary Care Trusts across the country and has supported many thousands of patients and will be applied throughout the NHS by 2008.

face to face WITH **CHRONIC DISEASE:**

MARIAM JOHN

" "I KNOW I

The failure to use available knowledge about chronic disease prevention and control endangers future generations.

CAN MAKE IT"

UNITED REPUBLIC
OF TANZANIA

MARIAM JOHN IS 13 YEARS OLD and already knows what she wants to be when she grows up – "a health minister can help others and wants everyone to be healthy," she says. "I have good grades, I know I can make it," she adds proudly.

In February 2005, soon after her knee started to swell to the point that it became difficult to walk, Mariam was diagnosed with bone cancer. She has been receiving chemotherapy and radiotherapy treatment since then – an almost unbearable experience. "I am willing to have my leg amputated if it can take my pain away," she concedes.

Name	Mariam John
Age	13
Country	United Republic of Tanzania
Diagnosis	Bone cancer

The day she was photographed, Mariam couldn't have her radio- therapy treatment owing to a power failure at the Dar es Salaam Cancer Institute. She had crawled painfully out of bed with her grandmother's help and been sitting crying in a wheelchair for half an hour, with nothing to support her swollen leg, before the news came.

Despite this terrible ordeal and great fatigue, Mariam remembers how to smile. Her best friend and classmate Maria is a fabulous supporter. "What cheers me up is when she writes me letters. She believes that I can be cured. I wish more people would think like her."

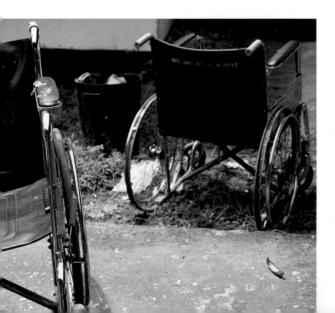

PLANNING STEP 3
Identify policy implementation steps

PROVIDE CARE ACROSS THE CONTINUUM

Ideally, health-care settings (primary, hospital or community-based) should provide complementary services that collectively span the care continuum from prevention through to rehabilitation and palliative care.

Implementation step	Suggested milestones
STEP 1 CORE	» Pain medication is provided as needed as part of end of life care.
STEP 2 EXPANDED	» Palliative services are provided to allow control of pain and other symptoms, and to permit death with dignity. » Community-based rehabilitation programmes are established.
STEP 3 DESIRABLE	» Multidisciplinary rehabilitation services are available.

PROMOTE MULTIDISCIPLINARY TEAMS

Multidisciplinary teams can consist of physicians, nurses, "expert patients" and others. Virtual teams – such as specialists linked to general practitioners by telephone – are increasingly common in rural or remote settings.

Implementation step	Suggested milestones
STEP 1 CORE	» Primary health-care workers are trained by specialists on chronic disease management and on when to refer to specialty care.
STEP 2 EXPANDED	» Remote links to specialists are established for rural health centres, and used for both consultation, referral and back-referral.
STEP 3 DESIRABLE	» Multidisciplinary primary health-care teams are organized, including, where possible, physicians, nurses, allied health professionals, and expert patients.

ENSURE THE HEALTH-CARE WORKFORCE HAS THE RIGHT COMPETENCIES

The health workforce is instrumental in stimulating, creating and maintaining improvements. Ministries of health should work with ministries of education and professional societies to ensure that the health workforce is taught the right skills to prepare them adequately for chronic disease prevention and management.

Continuing professional education allows the health workforce to develop skills after completion of training. Educational activities include courses, on-site follow-up and coaching, and regular assessments and feedback on progress. Medical, nursing and other health professional societies are valuable partners in the provision of continuing medical education.

Implementation step		Suggested milestones
STEP 1	**CORE**	» The health workforce, as part of its primary education, receives information and skills for chronic disease prevention and control.
STEP 2	**EXPANDED**	» On-the-job educational opportunities are provided.
STEP 3	**DESIRABLE**	» Continuing professional education on chronic disease prevention and management is mandated.

The private sector, civil society and international organizations

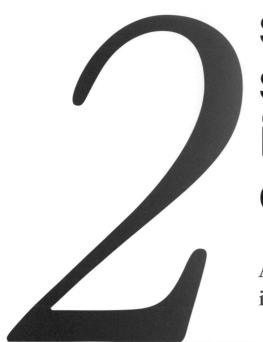

>> **Partnerships** among various groups, organizations and sectors are indispensable

>> **The private sector** is a natural partner in chronic disease prevention and control

>> **Civil society** plays a role that is distinct from that of governments and the private sector, and adds human and financial resources to a wide range of chronic disease prevention and control issues

>> **International organizations and donors** have important roles to play in the response to chronic disease

Any single organization or group is unlikely to have sufficient resources to tackle the complex public health issues related to the prevention and management of chronic diseases. The stepwise framework initiated by governments can be best implemented by working with some or all of the private sector, civil society and international organizations. This chapter outlines the ways in which such cooperation can be put into practice.

PARTNERSHIPS

Partnerships are collaborative relationships that bring together different parties to achieve a shared goal on the basis of a mutually agreed division of labour. Partnerships for health are indispensable. They offer all sectors new opportunities to work together in order to advance the greater public good. In order to be as effective as possible, they should work within the overall framework for prevention and control determined by the government (see previous chapter).

Working in partnership ensures synergies, avoids overlapping and duplication of activities, and prevents unnecessary or wasteful competition. Partnerships also provide a means of spreading the potential benefits of an initiative beyond what individual partners would achieve on their own, such as in Pakistan (see spotlight, left).

SUCCESS FACTORS

Partnerships work best when they:

» build on the unique roles of each partner;

» have specific objectives and expected outcomes;

» define clearly articulated roles and responsibilities for each partner;

» are implemented with the full agreement of all parties.

Developing and managing a successful partnership requires an appropriate organizational structure. There are different types of organizational models ranging from a simple affiliation to the creation of a separate and independent legal entity.

SPOTLIGHT
PUBLIC–PRIVATE PARTNERSHIP IN PAKISTAN

In Pakistan, the public–private tripartite collaborative arrangement, led by the nongovernmental organization Heartfile, with the Ministry of Health and the WHO Pakistan Office, has launched a partnership to develop and implement a national strategy for prevention and control of chronic diseases. The partnership has recently released a strategic framework for action, and work is under way on implementation.

Transparent linkages are being established to broaden the scope of this partnership with the private sector, including electronic media production houses, companies involved in the production, transport, storage and marketing of food items, private schools, road marking consultants, and industries with effluent discharge. Possibilities for partnerships with pharmaceutical companies are also being explored (8).

CONFLICTS OF INTEREST

Full disclosure of real or perceived conflicts of interest, both of individual staff and partner organizations, is required at the outset of partnership formation (it is not appropriate to work with some industries, such as tobacco and firearms).

NETWORKS

Networks are groups of individuals or organizations sharing a common interest, and in regular communication with each other to do their individual work more effectively. Two examples of different types of networks are given below.

SPOTLIGHT
CARMEN

The CARMEN (Conjunto de Acciones para la Reducción Multifactorial de Enfermedades No transmisibles) initiative aims to improve health in the Americas by reducing risk factors for chronic diseases. The main focus has been primary prevention of risk factors such as tobacco use, poor diet and physical inactivity.

The CARMEN network began with five countries/territories but has expanded to 16 (Argentina, Aruba, Brazil, Canada, Chile, Colombia, Costa Rica, Cuba, Curacao, El Salvador, Guatemala, Panama, Peru, Puerto Rico, Trinidad and Tobago, and Uruguay). Each has a national or sub-national action plan for chronic disease prevention and control, a focal point within the ministry of health to lead the activities, and usually a steering group to guide country-level activities. The network serves as a forum for advocacy, knowledge dissemination and management, and technical support and as an arena where directions, innovations and plans are made for continuous improvement of chronic disease prevention initiatives in the Americas.

The WHO Regional Office for the Americas serves as the secretariat for the CARMEN network, which has facilitated intraregional information sharing and collaboration. Similar networks have been initiated or are under development in other WHO regions.

SPOTLIGHT
PROCOR

ProCOR is an ongoing, e-mail and Internet-based open exchange. It aims to create a dynamic international forum where healthcare providers, researchers, public health workers and the general public can share information and participate in raising awareness about the epidemic of cardiovascular diseases in low and middle income countries.

Moderators screen incoming messages and post current research as well as clinical and public health information, thus ensuring the high scientific quality of the discussion (for more information see http://www.procor.org).

THE PRIVATE SECTOR

WORKPLACE HEALTH PROGRAMMES

Workplace initiatives to make healthy behaviour easier to achieve help to reduce people's risk of developing chronic diseases, while also benefiting employers. Most adults spend a significant portion of their time in a work environment and are often surrounded by peers who may influence their behaviour and attitudes.

Many interventions and programmes can be effectively implemented with limited resources and significant benefits to employees and employers, as illustrated by the Mobility India example (see spotlight, left). Healthy foods can be offered, workplaces and ventilation systems kept clean and tobacco-free, assistive devices installed, and physical activity promoted. Once basic programmes and options have been implemented or if more resources are available, employers can move on to initiate medium-term and long-term initiatives.

SPOTLIGHT
MOBILITY INDIA

Mobility India was established in 1994 to promote mobility in people with disabilities through awareness creation, advocacy, research, services, and integration of people with disabilities into society. Mobility India created the Millennium Building on Disability – the Mobility India Rehabilitation Research & Training Centre – as a model building to influence other organizations working in the field of disability and chronic conditions, and to increase understanding of accessibility issues. The building is friendly to all types of disabilities, and 40% of the staff have a disability.

Major features of the building include adequate ramps; Braille signs; tile floors with varied surfaces to guide people with visual impairments; accessible bathrooms, switchboards, and washbasins; a lift with auditory signals and an extra-sensitive door sensor; adequate and earmarked parking spaces; highly accessible hallways and workspaces with furniture kept in unchanged locations; and contrasting colour schemes and natural light for people with low vision.

The fact that Mobility India staff with personal experience of disabilities and chronic conditions are working in an accessible building has created a productive environment in which to work with confidence and dignity (9).

SPOTLIGHT
RIVER BLINDNESS

Merck Pharmaceutical Company discovered a new application for the drug Mectizan® (ivermectin) to prevent onchocerciasis, or river blindness, in the early 1980s. In 1987, it decided to donate as much as is needed to everyone who needs it for as long as it takes to eliminate the disease worldwide. Some 18 million people are infected with the parasitic worm, and 250 000 people are already irreparably blind from this disease. Mectizan® cannot restore lost sight but if it is taken early enough, it protects remaining vision. It kills the larvae responsible, and eliminates itching and damage to the eyes with just one dose per year, although infected people need to take Mectizan® for around 20 years. The Mectizan® donation programme has been a highly effective public health programme and serves as a possible model for tackling some future problems in international health.

PRODUCT DONATION/ PRICE REDUCTION PROGRAMMES

Affordable access to appropriate products is critical. The private sector can donate or offer them at affordable prices as part of a national plan, and help distribute products such as priority medications and medical devices. The success of the Mectizan® donation programme (see spotlight, left) is one example of such a programme.

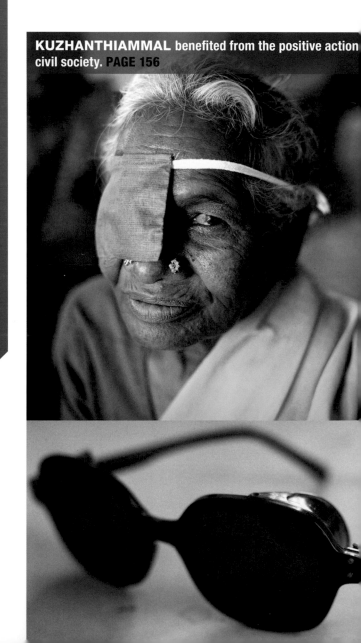

KUZHANTHIAMMAL benefited from the positive action civil society. **PAGE 156**

PRODUCT RESEARCH AND DEVELOPMENT

Many chronic diseases would benefit from the development of new medications or medical devices. The private sector has a significant role to play in closing these gaps, as do public–private partnerships, which can invest strategically to accelerate progress with regard to specific diseases. For example, biotechnology-based diagnostics can provide accurate and less expensive blood sugar and lipid assays, thereby eliminating the need for high technology laboratories and technologically trained personnel in the field. Alternatives to insulin delivery technologies, such as nasal sprays, could reduce the need for trained personnel, injection needles and refrigeration, and could revolutionize the management of diabetes. Affordable hearing aids (see spotlight, left) are another public health priority.

SPOTLIGHT
AFFORDABLE HEARING AIDS

WHO estimated in 2001 that over 90% of the 250 million people worldwide with disabling hearing impairment and deafness (of whom two thirds live in developing countries) would benefit from hearing aids. Current annual production of hearing aids provides approximately 33% of those needed in high income countries, but less than 3% of those needed in low and middle income countries.

Hearing aids in low and middle income countries range in pricc from US$ 200 to over US$ 500, prohibitive for the majority of people living there. Major companies are also reluctant to provide affordable hearing aids on a large scale because of their perceived lack of a sustainable market, and the lack of infrastructure to provide them.

Providing appropriate and affordable hearing aids and services worldwide would be a highly effective and cost-effective way to make a positive impact. Sustainable provision on a sufficiently large scale in low and middle income countries would also be crucial in terms of improving equity and access.

WHO has developed Guidelines for Hearing Aids and Services for Developing Countries as a tool for such programme development. The guidelines state that public–private partnerships between the governments of developing countries and hearing aid manufacturers are necessary. WHO and key stakeholders recently came together to set up an independent, collaborative network, called WWHearing (World-Wide Hearing Care for Developing Countries), to gather information on provision and need in developing countries, encourage appropriate, affordable hearing aids and services, stimulate public–private partnerships and promote projects for fitting, follow-up, repair and training. Countries in four WHO regions are in the process of setting up pilot studies to test the approach for these partnerships.

SPOTLIGHT
FOOD INDUSTRY ACCORD IN NEW ZEALAND

In 1999, new research showed that the health of New Zealand's people was affected more by unhealthy diet and physical inactivity combined than by other risk factors, including smoking. In response, the New Zealand Government developed a Healthy Eating – Healthy Action strategy (HEHA), with a wide range of stakeholders participating.

Members of the food and beverage industry are active HEHA stakeholders, and in September 2004 they launched a Food Industry Accord. All signatory food producers, distributors, retailers, marketers, advertisers and media outlets have acknowledged or publicized the fact that obesity is a major risk to public health, that the food industry has a role to play in tackling obesity, and that they will meet key objectives, such those aimed at reducing obesity, improving nutrition, and increasing physical activity. Actions and commitments resulting from the Food Industry Accord are being independently evaluated (*10*).

PRODUCT RESEARCH AND DEVELOPMENT – FOOD AND DRINKS

Initiatives by the food and drink industries to reduce the fat, sugar and salt content of processed foods as well as portion sizes, to increase choice, and to review current marketing practices could accelerate health gains worldwide. Recommendations of the WHO Global Strategy on Diet, Physical Activity and Health to the food and drink industries include the following:

» limit the levels of saturated fats, trans-fatty acids, free sugars and salt in existing products;

» continue to develop and provide affordable, healthy and nutritious choices to consumers;

» consider introducing new products with better nutritional value (*11*).

Many companies have already made some modifications to product composition by lowering portion sizes and altering contents. Some have introduced low/reduced fat and low salt products, as well as offering fruit and salads in fast food outlets. These actions have been taken voluntarily by companies, although perhaps accelerated by the broader policy environment.

SPOTLIGHT
REDUCING SALT INTAKE
IN THE UNITED KINGDOM

In November 2003 a "Salt Summit" in the UK brought together departmental health ministers, the Chief Medical Officer, the chair of the Food Standards Agency, food retailers, producers, caterers, and health and consumer groups to discuss plans to reduce salt in foods to meet the government's target of reducing salt consumption in the population from 9.5 g to an average of 6 g per person per day by 2010.

The summit concluded that reduction programmes were taking place on a broad front with action at different stages between different companies and sectors. However, further work was needed to meet the reduction target. A joint programme of work has been agreed between the Department of Health and the Food Standards Agency, following meetings with industry and the submission of their plans. By February 2005, around 65 key food industry organizations met government officials to discuss salt reduction plans, resulting in 52 commitments from across all sectors of the food industry.

In September 2004, the Food Standards Agency launched a high-profile consumer awareness campaign on salt. The tracking research is now showing a steady increase in the number of people who recognize that they might have a problem with too much salt in their diet and who are now trying to cut down. Between August 2004 and January 2005 there was:

- a 32% increase in people claiming to be making a special effort to cut down on salt;
- an increase of 31% in those who look at labelling to find out salt content;
- a 27% increase in those who say that salt content would affect their decision to buy a product "all of the time".

The next stage of the programme of work with industry will include the following:

- Establishing targets for specific categories of foods, especially those making the greatest contribution to population salt intakes; proposed targets have been identified following discussion with the industry and a public consultation is being held prior to publication of the targets in November 2005.
- Obtaining further long-term plans with specific measurable stepwise commitments to salt reduction capable of delivering the Government's target of 6g average daily intake by 2010, as well as securing clear data from all relevant organizations to ensure that salt reduction claims can be verified.
- Focusing on securing further salt reductions particularly in the cereal and meat, pizzas, ready meals and sandwich product categories (these make the biggest contributions to adult salt intakes in the UK).
- Developing a clear programme of work for the catering sector and public procurement, including specific guidelines for salt reduction, in consultation with the key stakeholders.

At the global level, WHO is convening a series of discussions with food and drink companies, retailers and nongovernmental organizations to encourage more action, although such activities are sometimes best coordinated and more efficiently managed at the regional or sub-regional level. For example, the European Commission recently launched a Platform for Action on voluntary but measurable reductions in salt, sugar and fat content and improved product information for consumers. National regulators and regional organizations have also established guidelines and targets for lowering the fat, salt and sugar content of processed foods. The Food Standards Agency in the United Kingdom, for example, has developed a national plan of action including targets for salt reduction (see spotlight, left).

OTHER ROLES

Other roles for the private sector include information and experience sharing. The private sector possesses essential and specialized skills that are valuable for chronic disease prevention and control. For example, expertise in marketing, advertising and brand promotion could be offered to strengthen public awareness and education campaigns.

Charitable giving is another way in which the private sector can contribute to chronic disease prevention and control.

The media and entertainment industry can use programming, media access and celebrity figures to deliver key messages about chronic diseases.

INDIA
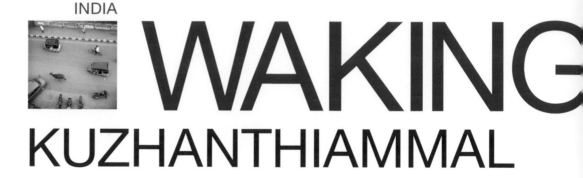

WAKING
KUZHANTHIAMMAL

KUZHANTHIAMMAL BEGAN TO WORRY TWO YEARS AGO when a white film clouding her left eye would not clear away. It was keeping her from working on her land and taking care of her teenage granddaughter. As for many poor Indians, a visit to hospital was out of reach, for both economic and geographical reasons.

Soon after the first symptoms appeared, Kuzhanthiammal heard of an eye diagnostic camp that was taking place at a nearby village. She decided to attend, and within a few minutes was diagnosed and registered for free cataract surgery at the Madwai Aravind Eye Hospital the following week.

Name	Kuzhanthiammal
Age	67
Country	India
Diagnosis	Cataract

The programme even covered transport costs. "A bus picked me up with seven other cataract patients and drove us to the hospital," she says. Some 70% of Aravind's eye patients are charity cases; the 30% who are paying customers support these free sight-restoring operations. The hospital also sells abroad three quarters of the lenses it produces, to help finance its activities.

Now 67 years old, Kuzhanthiammal successfully underwent surgery on her other eye a few months ago. "These artificial lenses are a miracle. It's like waking up with your problems gone," she joyfully explains.

156

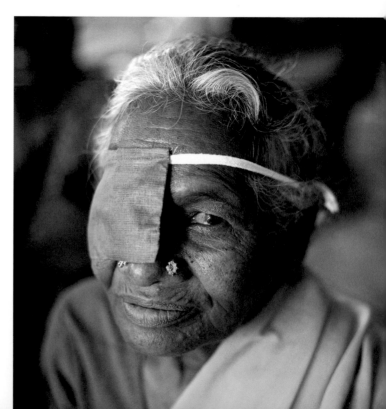

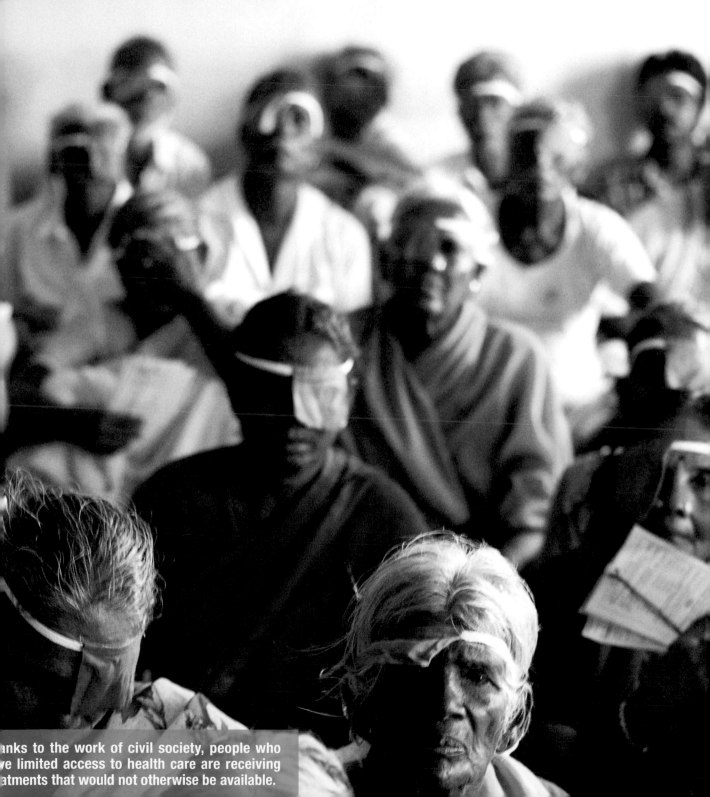

JP TO VISION

anks to the work of civil society, people who
e limited access to health care are receiving
atments that would not otherwise be available.

CIVIL SOCIETY

The term civil society refers to a broad array of organizations that are essentially private and outside the institutional structures of government, but at the same time are not primarily commercial and do not exist principally to distribute profits to their directors or owners. Civil society includes organizations such as registered charities, nongovernmental organizations, professional societies and advocacy groups.

These and other organizations add human and financial resources to a wide range of chronic disease prevention and control issues (see spotlight, left). In addition, they occupy a role that is distinct from that of governments and the private sector. In many cases, civil society works parallel to or in partnership with government and the private sector. Sometimes, civil society takes the lead on public health issues. It can stimulate efforts by:

» supporting the wide dissemination of information;

» promoting public debate;

» leading grass-roots mobilization;

» encouraging policy-makers to translate evidence into action;

» organizing campaigns and events that stimulate action by all stakeholders;

» improving health-care service delivery;

» creating partnerships among stakeholders.

SPOTLIGHT
WORLD HEART DAY AND WORLD DIABETES DAY

One of the ways in which nongovernmental organizations draw attention to issues is by means of annual health days. The World Heart Federation, for example, initiated the World Heart Day programme in the year 2000 to increase awareness of cardiovascular disease prevention and control, particularly in low and middle income countries. World Heart Day is celebrated on the last Sunday of September each year. This programme is co-sponsored by WHO and UNESCO and is now recognized by UNICEF. In 2000, 63 countries and 103 World Heart Federation member organizations participated by running national programmes. By 2004, more than 100 countries were involved and 312 members and partners ran national activities. UNESCO distributed the World Heart Day materials to its 175 regional offices and to 7500 schools. WHO's Regional Office for Africa distributed materials to 46 African countries and has been directly involved in building successful national programmes. An audience of 365 million readers, viewers and listeners was reached internationally (in the English language alone).

Similarly, the International Diabetes Federation celebrates World Diabetes Day annually on 14 November. The day is marked worldwide by the 185 member associations of the Federation in more than 145 countries, as well as by other associations and organizations, health-care professionals and individuals with an interest in diabetes. The Federation produces a variety of support materials for its member associations which in turn distribute them to people with diabetes and their families, the general public, health-care professionals and the media, as well as to local and national decision-makers.

INTERNATIONAL ORGANIZATIONS

International organizations, including United Nations agencies, donors and development banks have crucial roles to play. Some of their work is described in this report. Coordinated action is needed among the organizations of the United Nations system, intergovernmental bodies, nongovernmental organizations, professional associations, research institutions and private sector entities.

In particular, the World Health Organization has received several global mandates from its governing bodies to take action on chronic disease prevention and control, such as the Global Strategy for the Prevention and Control of Noncommunicable Diseases, the Global Strategy on Diet, Physical Activity and Health, and the WHO Framework Convention on Tobacco Control. Many relevant mandates have also been adopted by WHO regional governing bodies. These provide the basis for taking international action in support of regional and national efforts to prevent and control chronic diseases and their common risk factors.

CONCLUSION

Taking action to halt and turn back the rising chronic disease pandemic is a pressing challenge for the field of global public health. Fortunately, the effective and feasible strategies for doing so already exist. The global goal of saving 36 million lives by the year 2015 can be achieved with urgent, coordinated action.

A range of effective interventions for chronic disease prevention and control exist, and many countries have already made major reductions in chronic disease death rates through their implementation.

Everyone has a role to play in advancing the agenda. In low income countries, it is vital that supportive policies are put in place now to reduce risks and curb the epidemics before they take hold. In countries with established chronic disease problems, additional measures are needed not only to prevent the diseases through population wide and individual risk reduction but also to manage illness and prevent complications.

Taking up the challenge for chronic disease prevention and control, especially in the context of competing priorities, requires courage and ambition. On the other hand, the failure to use available knowledge about chronic disease prevention and control is unjustified, and recklessly endangers future generations. There is simply no excuse for allowing chronic diseases to continue taking millions of lives each year when the scientific understanding of how to prevent these deaths is available now. The agenda is broad and bold, but the way forward is clear.

REFERENCES

1. *STEPS: a framework for surveillance.* Geneva, World Health Organization, 2003 (http://www.who.int/ncd_surveillance/en/steps_framework_dec03.pdf, accessed 5 July 2005).

2. Wang L, Kong L, Wu F, Bai Y, Burton R. Preventing chronic diseases in China. *Lancet* (in press).

3. Tonga Ministry of Health. *A National Strategy to Prevent and Control Noncommunicable Diseases in Tonga.* Nuku' Alofa: Tonga MOH, 2003.

4. Mohan V, Shanthirani CS, Deepa R. Glucose intolerance (diabetes and IGT) in a selected south Indian population with special reference to family history, obesity and life style factors – The Chennai Urban Population Study (CUPS 14). *Journal of the Association of Physicians of India*, 2003, 51:771–777.

5. Doak C. Large-scale interventions and programmes addressing nutrition-related chronic diseases and obesity: examples from 14 countries. *Public Health Nutrition*, 2002, 5(1A):275–277.

6. Xia SC, Zhang XW, Xu SY, Tang SM, Yu SH, Aldinger C et al. Creating health-promoting schools in China with a focus on nutrition. *Health Promotion International*, 2004, 19:409–418.

7. Glasauer P, Aldinger C, Yu SH, Xia SC, Tang SM. Nutrition as an entry point for health-promoting schools: lessons from China. *Food, Nutrition and Agriculture*, 2003, 33:27–33.

8. Nishtar S. The National Action Plan for the Prevention and Control of Non-communicable Diseases and Health Promotion in Pakistan – Prelude and finale. *Journal of the Pakistan Medical Association*, 2004, 54(12 Suppl. 3):S1-8.

9. Mobility India (http://www.mobility-india.org/, accessed 5 July 2005).

10. *Healthy eating – healthy action, oranga kai – oranga pumau. Implementation plan: 2004–2010.* Wellington, Ministry of Health, 2004 (http://www.moh.govt.nz/moh.nsf/ accessed 5 July 2005).

11. *Global strategy on diet, physical activity and health.* World Health Assembly resolution WHA57.17. Geneva, World Health Organization, 2004 (http://www.who.int/gb/ebwha/pdf_files/WHA57/A57_R17-en.pdf, accessed 5 July 2005).

ANNEXES

1 Methods for projections of mortality and burden of disease to 2015

WHO has prepared updated projections of trends for mortality and burden of disease between 2002 and 2015 using methods similar to those used in the original Global Burden of Disease (GBD) study (1). A set of relatively simple models was used to project future health trends under various scenarios, based largely on projections of economic and social development, and using the historically observed relationships of these to cause-specific mortality rates. The data inputs for the projection models have been updated to take account of the greater number of countries reporting death registration data to WHO, particularly developing countries, and to take into account other recently developed projection models on HIV/AIDS and other conditions where appropriate, as well as tobacco epidemics.

A BRIEF OVERVIEW OF THE METHODS AND ASSUMPTIONS

Rather than attempt to model the effects of the many separate direct determinants or risk factors for disease from the limited data that are available, the GBD methodology considered a limited number of socioeconomic variables: average income per capita, measured as gross domestic product (GDP) per capita; average number of years of schooling in adults, referred to as "human capital"; and time, a proxy measure for the impact of technological change on health status. This latter variable captures the effects of accumulating knowledge and technological development, allowing the implementation

of more cost-effective health interventions, both preventive and curative, at constant levels of income and human capital (2).

These socioeconomic variables show clear historical relationships with mortality rates, and may be regarded as indirect, or distal, determinants of health. In addition, a fourth variable, tobacco use, was included in the projections for cancers, cardiovascular diseases and chronic respiratory diseases, because of its overwhelming importance in determining trends for these causes. Tobacco use was measured in terms of "smoking intensity" – that component of observed lung cancer mortality that is attributable to tobacco smoking (3).

For the projections reported here, death rates for all major causes excluding HIV/AIDS were related to these four variables using historical death registration data for 107 countries between 1950 and 2002 (4). Death rates were then projected using World Bank projections of GDP per capita, WHO projections of human capital, and smoking intensity projections based on historical patterns of tobacco use and further adjusted for recent regional trends in tobacco consumption where appropriate.

Separate projections for HIV/AIDS mortality were prepared by UNAIDS and WHO, under a scenario in which coverage with antiretroviral drugs reaches 80% by 2012, remaining constant beyond that year, and in which there are no changes to current transmission rates due to increased prevention efforts. Projected tuberculosis mortality rates were modified in regions with high HIV prevalence, owing to the expected interaction of tuberculosis and HIV. Because a substantial proportion of diabetes mortality is attributable to overweight and obesity (*5*), a separate projection model for diabetes mortality was developed using WHO projection of trends in body mass index distributions from 2000 to 2010. Similarly, projections of mortality for chronic respiratory diseases were adjusted for projected changes in smoking intensity.

The original GBD projections assumed that the changes in death rates associated with income growth and time in countries with death registration data, mostly medium and high income countries, would also apply in low income countries. The new projections for low income countries were based on the observed relationships for a data set consisting of 3468 country-years of observation where income per capita was less than $10 000 per year. Additionally, observed regional trends in child mortality from 1990 to 2002 were compared with those predicted by the projection model for low income countries. As a result, the regression coefficient for time was set to zero for sub-Saharan Africa, and to 25% of its original value for other low income countries.

The WHO projections of mortality rates to 2015, together with UN medium variant assumptions for fertility rates and migration rates (*6*), were also used to prepare consistent population projections for all regions. The projected global population in 2015 was 7.1 billion compared to the UN medium variant projection of 7.2 billion, reflecting somewhat higher adult death rates in the WHO mortality projections.

PROJECTIONS FOR COUNTRIES

Projections were carried out at country level, but aggregated into regional or income groups for presentation of results, apart from the projections for nine selected countries included in this report. Baseline estimates at country level for 2002 were derived from the GBD analyses published in *The World Health Report 2004* (*7*). Mortality estimates were based on analysis of latest available national information on levels of mortality and cause distributions as at late 2003. Incidence, prevalence, duration and severity estimates for conditions were based on the GBD analyses for the relevant epidemiological subregion, together with national and sub-national level information available to WHO. These baseline estimates represent the best estimates of WHO,

based on the evidence available in mid-2004, rather than the official estimates of Member States, and have been computed using standard categories and methods to maximize cross-national comparability.

Initial WHO estimates and technical explanations were sent to Member States for comment in 2003, and comments or additional information incorporated where possible. Country-specific projections were shared with relevant WHO country offices and Member States in advance of publication.

LIMITATIONS

By their very nature, projections of the future are highly uncertain and need to be interpreted with caution. Three limitations are briefly discussed: uncertainties in the baseline data on levels and trends in cause-specific mortality, the "business as usual" assumptions, and the use of a relatively simple model based largely on projections of economic and social development.

For regions with limited death registration data, such as the Eastern Mediterranean Region, sub-Saharan Africa and parts of Asia and the Pacific, there is considerable uncertainty in estimates of deaths by cause associated with the use of partial information on levels of mortality from sources such as the Demographic and Health Surveys, and from the use of cause-specific mortality estimates for causes such as HIV/AIDS, malaria, tuberculosis and vaccine-preventable diseases (*8*). The GBD analyses have attempted to use all available sources of information, together with an explicit emphasis on internal consistency, to develop consistent and comprehensive estimates of deaths and disease burden by cause, age, sex and region.

The projections of burden are not intended as forecasts of what will happen in the future but as projections of current and past trends, based on certain explicit assumptions and on observed historical relationships between development and mortality levels and patterns. The methods used base the disease burden projections largely on broad mortality projections driven to a large extent by World Bank projections of future growth in income per capita in different regions of the world. As a result, it is important to interpret the projections with a degree of caution commensurate with their uncertainty, and to remember that they represent a view of the future explicitly resulting from the baseline data, choice of models, and the assumptions made. Uncertainty in projections has been addressed not through an attempt to estimate uncertainty ranges, but through preparation of pessimistic and optimistic projections under alternate sets of input assumptions.

The results depend strongly on the assumption that future mortality trends in poor countries will have the same relationship to economic and social development as has occurred in higher income countries in the recent past. If this assumption is not correct, then the projections for low income countries will be over-optimistic in the rate of decline of communicable and noncommunicable diseases. The projections have also not taken explicit account of trends in major risk factors apart from tobacco smoking and, to a limited extent, overweight and obesity. If broad trends in risk factors are for worsening of risk exposures with development, rather than the improvements observed in recent decades in many high income countries, then again the projections for low and middle income countries presented here will be too optimistic.

THE GLOBAL GOAL

The global goal for chronic diseases, proposed in this report, was modelled in terms of an additional 2% annual decline in chronic disease death rates from 2006 to 2015. Annual rates of change in age and sex specific death rates for all chronic disease causes were calculated for the mortality projections from 2005 to 2015 and then adjusted by subtraction of an additional 2% per annum. Death rates for the years 2006 to 2015 were then recomputed using the adjusted annual trends for age/sex-specific rates. Note that the final death rates for chronic diseases in 2015 under the bold goal scenario will be substantially lower than the base projections, since the additional 2% annual declines are cumulative.

FURTHER INFORMATION

Interested readers can visit the WHO web site at http://www.who.int/evidence/bod, where the following information is available:

» mortality and burden of disease estimates for 2002 for WHO regions and for countries grouped by income level;

» downloadable working papers on the data sources, methodology and tools used in assessment of mortality and burden of disease for 2002;

» a downloadable technical paper giving a detailed description of the data inputs, methods and results for the projections of mortality and burden of disease;

» links to other publications and results relating to the WHO projections.

REFERENCES

1. Murray CJL, Lopez AD. Alternative projections of mortality and disability by cause 1990-2020: Global Burden of Disease Study. *Lancet*, 1997, 349:1498–1504.

2. Murray C JL, Lopez AD. Alternative visions of the future: projecting mortality and disability, 1990-2020. In: Murray CJL, Lopez AD, eds. *The global burden of disease: a comprehensive assessment of mortality and disability from diseases, injuries and risk factors in 1990 and projected to 2020.* Cambridge, MA, Harvard School of Public Health on behalf of the World Health Organization and the World Bank, 1996 (Global Burden of Disease and Injury Series, Vol. I).

3. Peto R, Lopez AD, Boreham J, Thun M, Heath C. Mortality from tobacco in developed countries: indirect estimation from national vital statistics. *Lancet*, 1992, 339:1268–1278.

4. Mathers CD, Ma Fat D, Inoue M, Rao C, Lopez AD. Counting the dead and what they died from: an assessment of the global status of cause of death data. *Bulletin of the World Health Organization*, 2005, 83:171–177.

5. James WPT, Jackson-Leach R, Ni Mhurchu C, Kalamara E, Shayeghi M, Rigby NJ et al. Overweight and obesity (high body mass index). In: Ezzati M, Lopez AD, Rodgers A, Murray CJL, eds. *Comparative quantification of health risks: global and regional burden of disease attributable to selected major risk factors.* Geneva, World Health Organization, 2004 (http://www.who.int/publications/cra, accessed 27 July 2005).

6. *World population prospects – the 2002 revision.* New York, NY, United Nations Population Division, 2003.

7 *The world health report 2004 – Changing history.* Geneva, World Health Organization, 2004 (http://www.who.int/whr, accessed 27 July 2005).

8. Mathers CD, Bernard C, Iburg KM, Inoue M, Ma Fat D, Shibuya K et al. *Global burden of disease in 2002: data sources, methods and results.* Geneva, World Health Organization, 2003 (GPE Discussion Paper No. 54).

2 WHO regions

AFRICA	AMERICAS	SOUTH-EAST A
Algeria	Antigua and Barbuda	Bangladesh
Angola	Argentina	Bhutan
Benin	Bahamas	Democratic People's Republic of Korea
Botswana	Barbados	India
Burkina Faso	Belize	Indonesia
Burundi	Bolivia	Maldives
Cameroon	Brazil	Myanmar
Cape Verde	Canada	Nepal
Central African Republic	Chile	Sri Lanka
Chad	Colombia	Thailand
Comoros	Costa Rica	Timor-Leste
Congo	Cuba	
Côte d'Ivoire	Dominica	
Democratic Republic of the Congo	Dominican Republic	
Equatorial Guinea	Ecuador	
Eritrea	El Salvador	
Ethiopia	Grenada	
Gabon	Guatemala	
Gambia	Guyana	
Ghana	Haiti	
Guinea	Honduras	
Guinea-Bissau	Jamaica	
Kenya	Mexico	
Lesotho	Nicaragua	
Liberia	Panama	
Madagascar	Paraguay	
Malawi	Peru	
Mali	Saint Kitts and Nevis	
Mauritania	Saint Lucia	
Mauritius	Saint Vincent and the Grenadines	
Mozambique	Suriname	
Namibia	Trinidad and Tobago	
Niger	United States of America	
Nigeria	Uruguay	
Rwanda	Venezuela (Bolivarian Republic of)	
Sao Tome and Principe		
Senegal		
Seychelles		
Sierra Leone		
South Africa		
Swaziland		
Togo		
Uganda		
United Republic of Tanzania		
Zambia		
Zimbabwe		

OPE	EASTERN MEDITERRANEAN	WESTERN PACIFIC
a	Afghanistan	Australia
a	Bahrain	Brunei Darussalam
'a	Djibouti	Cambodia
a	Egypt	China
ijan	Iran (Islamic Republic of)	Cook Islands
s	Iraq	Fiji
n	Jordan	Japan
and Herzegovina	Kuwait	Kiribati
a	Lebanon	Lao People's Democratic Republic
a	Libyan Arab Jamahiriya	Malaysia
.	Morocco	Marshall Islands
Republic	Oman	Micronesia (Federated States of)
rk	Pakistan	Mongolia
a	Qatar	Nauru
d	Saudi Arabia	New Zealand
	Somalia	Niue
a	Sudan	Palau
ny	Syrian Arab Republic	Papua New Guinea
.	Tunisia	Philippines
ry	United Arab Emirates	Republic of Korea
d	Yemen	Samoa
		Singapore
		Solomon Islands
		Tonga
nstan		Tuvalu
stan		Vanuatu
		Viet Nam
nia		
bourg		
o		
lands		
y		
al		
ic of Moldova		
ia		
n Federation		
arino		
and Montenegro		
ia		
a		
n		
rland		
an		
mer Yugoslav ic of Macedonia		
enistan		
e		
Kingdom		
stan		

3

World Bank income groupings

For operational and analytical purposes, the World Bank's main criterion for classifying economies is gross national income (GNI) per capita. Based on its GNI per capita, every economy is classified as low income, middle income (subdivided into lower middle and upper middle), or high income.

Categories for this report were based on the income categories published in *World development indicators 2003*, Washington, DC, World Bank, 2003. Economies were divided according to 2001 GNI per capita, calculated using the World Bank Atlas method. The groups are: low income, US$ 745 or less; lower middle income, US$ 746–2975; upper middle income, US$ 2976–9205; and high income, US$ 9206 or more.

COUNTRIES, AREAS AND TERRITORIE

HIGH INCOME	UPPER MIDDLE INC
Andorra	American Samoa
Aruba	Antigua and Barbuda
Australia	Argentina
Austria	Barbados
Bahamas	Botswana
Bahrain	Brazil
Belgium	Chile
Bermuda	Costa Rica
Brunei Darussalam	Croatia
Canada	Czech Republic
Cayman Islands	Dominica
Channel Islands	Estonia
Cyprus	Gabon
Denmark	Grenada
Faroe Islands	Hungary
Finland	Isle of Man
France	Latvia
French Polynesia	Lebanon
Germany	Libyan Arab Jamahiriya
Greece	Lithuania
Greenland	Malaysia
Guam	Malta
Iceland	Mauritius
Ireland	Mexico
Israel	Oman
Italy	Palau
Japan	Panama
Kuwait	Poland
Liechtenstein	Puerto Rico
Luxembourg	Saint Kitts and Nevis
Monaco	Saint Lucia
Netherlands	Saudi Arabia
Netherlands Antilles	Seychelles
New Caledonia	Slovakia
New Zealand	Trinidad and Tobago
Northern Mariana Islands	Uruguay
Norway	Venezuela (Bolivarian Republi
Portugal	
Qatar	
Republic of Korea	
San Marino	
Singapore	
Slovenia	
Spain	
Sweden	
Switzerland	
United Arab Emirates	
United Kingdom	
United States of America	
United States Virgin Islands	

VER MIDDLE INCOME

a

a

s

a

a and Herzegovina

ria

Verde

bia

ti

ican Republic

or

vador

mala

a

uras

slamic Republic of)

ca

n

hstan

ti

ves

all Islands

nesia (Federated States of)

co

bia

uay

pines

nia

an Federation

Vincent and the Grenadines

a

a and Montenegro

Africa

nka

ame

land

Arab Republic

nd

rmer Yugoslav Republic of Macedonia

a

a

y

nenistan

tu

Bank and Gaza

LOW INCOME

Afghanistan	Liberia
Angola	Madagascar
Armenia	Malawi
Azerbaijan	Mali
Bangladesh	Mauritania
Benin	Mongolia
Bhutan	Mozambique
Burkina Faso	Myanmar
Burundi	Nepal
Cambodia	Nicaragua
Cameroon	Niger
Central African Republic	Nigeria
Chad	Pakistan
Comoros	Papua New Guinea
Congo	Republic of Moldova
Côte d'Ivoire	Rwanda
Democratic People's Republic of Korea	Sao Tome and Principe
Democratic Republic of the Congo	Senegal
Equatorial Guinea	Sierra Leone
Eritrea	Solomon Islands
Ethiopia	Somalia
Gambia	Sudan
Georgia	Tajikistan
Ghana	Timor-Leste
Guinea	Togo
Guinea-Bissau	Uganda
Haiti	Ukraine
India	United Republic of Tanzania
Indonesia	Uzbekistan
Kenya	Viet Nam
Kyrgyzstan	Yemen
Lao People's Democratic Republic	Zambia
Lesotho	Zimbabwe

4 Economic analysis methods

For the economic analyses of this report, three approaches were adopted:

1. systematic review on chronic disease costs of illness;

2. elucidation of the human capital impact of chronic diseases through their impact on labour supply – the Solow growth model using the Cobb-Douglas function;

3. elucidation of the impact of chronic diseases on and growth in economic welfare – the full-income approach.

Estimation of the economic impact was based on projections to 2015 for nine countries: Brazil, Canada, China, India, Nigeria, Pakistan, the Russian Federation, the United Kingdom and the United Republic of Tanzania. The focus was on heart disease, stroke and diabetes.

THE GROWTH (COBB-DOUGLAS) MODEL

The Cobb-Douglas function (equation 1) was combined with the capital accumulation function (equation 2) to estimate the long-run impact of chronic diseases on economic growth for these countries.

$$Y_{it} = r \, A_{it} K_{it}^{\alpha} L_{it}^{1-\alpha} \qquad (1)$$

Where:
Y = national (production) income – GDP pc
K = capital accumulation
L = labour inputs
α = Elasticity of Y with respect to K
$1 - \alpha$ = elasticity of Y with respect to L
i = countries
t = time period
r = adjustment factor (Cuddington et al., 1992)

Note that $\alpha + (1-\alpha)$ = unity, i.e. constant returns to scale.

$$K_{it} = sY_{it} - xC_{it} + (1-\delta)K_{i(t-1)} \qquad (2)$$

Where:
Y, K, *i* and *t* are as defined in above
s = savings rate
C = cost of treating illness
x = proportion of C funded from savings
δ = depreciation

APPROACH TO ELUCIDATION

Three main approaches were initially considered: (1) econometric estimation and projections; (2) econometric estimation and calibration; and (3) straightforward calibration using information on variables from various sources. The third approach was adopted for this phase of work because of data availability issues and time constraints. However, options 1 and 2 will be pursed as part of the ongoing work in this area, and as a follow-up to the report.

DATA AND DATA SOURCES

Projected gross domestic product (GDP) data were obtained from the World Bank and converted to GDP per worker as all other variable input. Capital per worker was obtained from Easterly & Levine (*1*). Information on the impact of chronic diseases on labour supply was obtained from the population and mortality projections of the Global Burden of Disease Unit of WHO. Costs of treating chronic diseases were obtained from WHO sources. Historical savings rates, depreciation, were obtained from the World Bank Development Index database.

For the base case estimated, proportion of cost of treating illness funded from savings was set at 10%. Region-specific elasticities of Y with respect to K were obtained from Senhadji (*2*). There was difficulty in obtaining data for capital accumulation in the Russian Federation; this was then set to the average of countries. All these variables were then subjected to sensitivity analysis.

THE FULL-INCOME MODEL

The full-income (FI) approach captures the value of changes in population health in the assessment of "economic welfare" (*3, 4*). The welfare value of deaths or changes in life expectancy from disease, estimated through the Value of Statistical Life (VSL) (Value of a Life Year (VLY)) nexus is added to changes in annual GDP per capita. For example, if Δp = change in the probability of dying within a given period say 2005–2015, and VSL = 100 times GDP per capita the welfare loss from mortality = (Δp x 100) X GDP per capita X (proportion of adults in the population). Suppose Δp = 0.4% and proportion of adults in pop = 50%, then welfare loss = 0.4 X GDP X 0.5 = 20% of GDP per capita. That is, GDP per capita would have been 20% of the actual GDP per capita. This would correspond to a rate of decrease in economic welfare due to mortality increase of 2% per annum. This approach, which may seem more complete than the previous approaches, does not account for the total value of the changes in health. It is, however, useful in that it demonstrates fuller returns to investment in health compared to the above approaches. Estimation should be of interest to country development strategists and policy-makers in the health and finance sectors, and also useful for international comparison.

MODEL PROGRAMMING AND ELUCIDATION

Microsoft Excel was used to programme the relationships in the equations from 2002 to 2015. The model was programmed to compute output if there were no deaths due to chronic disease (the counterfactual) against output given the projected deaths from chronic disease on an annual basis. This procedure was then repeated for estimating the global goal of an additional 2% annual reduction in chronic disease death rates over and above baseline projections, over 10 years from 2006 to 2015.

All the variables in the Cobb-Douglas model were subjected to univariate and multivariate analysis (Monte Carlo) using Crystal Ball software.

1. Easterly W, Levine R. What have we learned from a decade of empirical research on growth? It's not factor accumulation: stylized facts and growth models. *World Bank Economic Review*, 2001, 15:177–219.
2. Senhadji A. Sources of economic growth: an extensive accounting exercise. IMF Institute, *IMF Staff Papers*, 2000, 47:129–158 (http://www.imf.org/external/Pubs/FT/staffp/2000/00-01/pdf/senhadji.pdf, accessed 2 August 2005).
3. Nordhaus WD. *The health of nations: the contribution of improved health to living standards*. New Haven, CT, Yale University, 2002 (Cowles Foundation Discussion Paper, No. 1355).
4. Usher D. An imputation to the measure of economic growth for changes in life expectancy. In: Moss M, ed. *The measurement of economic and social performance*. New York, NY, Columbia University Press, 1973:193–226.

5 The WHO-CHOICE method

The CHOICE (**CHO**osing **I**nterventions that are **C**ost-**E**ffective) project was developed by WHO in 1998. The objective is to provide policy-makers with evidence on which to base decisions regarding interventions and programmes, given the need to provide the best health gains possible with available resources. WHO-CHOICE reports the costs and effects of a wide range of health interventions in 14 epidemiological sub-regions (world divisions made based on geographical location and epidemiological profiles). The results of these cost–effectiveness analyses are assembled in regional databases, which policy-makers can adapt to their specific country setting.

According to the cost–effectiveness results, interventions can be grouped into three categories:

COST–EFFECTIVENESS CATEGORY	DEFINITION
Very cost-effective	Interventions that avert each DALY at a cost less than gross domestic product per head.
Cost-effective	Interventions that avert each DALY at a cost between one and three times gross domestic product per head.
Not cost-effective	Interventions that avert each DALY at a cost higher than three times gross domestic product per head.

Interested readers can visit the WHO CHOICE web site at http://www.who.int/choice where the following information is available:

» cost–effectiveness results of the interventions evaluated for the 14 world sub-regions;

» a list of countries in the 14 sub-regions used for the WHO-CHOICE analysis;

» downloadable background papers on the methodology and tools used in conducting the WHO-CHOICE cost–effectiveness analyses;

» detailed region-specific demographic data and list of input variables, including prices and quantities, exchange rates, price multipliers and other key reference material for conducting cost–effectiveness analyses;

» a brief description on the WHO guide to cost–effectiveness analysis (1), the theoretical and practical compendium on CHOICE methodology.

1. Tan Torres T, Baltussen RM, Adam T, Hutubessy RC, Acharya A, Evans DB et al. *Making choices in health: WHO guide to cost–effectiveness analysis.* Geneva, World Health Organization, 2003.

Acknowledgements

Preventing chronic diseases: a vital investment was produced with the input, guidance and assistance of many colleagues. Valuable material, help and advice were received from policy advisers to the Director-General and many technical staff at WHO headquarters, regional directors and members of their staff, WHO country representatives and country office staff. These contributions have been vital to the project, both in creating and enriching the report.

The production of this publication was made possible through the generous financial support of the Government of Canada, the Government of Norway and the Government of the United Kingdom.

EDITOR-IN-CHIEF
Robert Beaglehole,
   Director, Department of Chronic
   Diseases and Health Promotion

MANAGING EDITOR
JoAnne Epping-Jordan,
   Senior Programme Adviser,
   Department of Chronic Diseases
   and Health Promotion

CORE COORDINATION TEAM
Robert Beaglehole
JoAnne Epping-Jordan
Elmira Adenova
Stéfanie Durivage
Amanda Marlin
Karen McCaffrey
Alexandra Munro
Caroline Savitzky
Kristin Thompson

ADVISORY GROUP
Catherine Le Galès-Camus
Andres de Francisco
Stephen Matlin
Jane McElligott
Christine McNab
Isabel Mortara
Margaret Peden
Thomson Prentice

Laura Sminkey
Ian Smith
Nigel Unwin
Janet Voûte

ADMINISTRATIVE AND SECRETARIAL SUPPORT
Elmira Adenova
Virgie Largado-Ferri
Rachel Pedersen

EXTERNAL EXPERT REVIEWERS
WHO gratefully acknowledges the following people for reviewing draft versions of the report. Expert reviewers do not necessarily endorse the full contents of the final version.

Olusoji Adeyi, World Bank
Julien Bogousslavsky, International Stroke Society
Debbie Bradshaw, Medical Research Council of South Africa
Jonathan Betz Brown, Kaiser Permanente, USA
Robert Burton, National Cancer Control Initiative, Australia
Catherine Coleman, ProCOR, Lown Cardiovascular Research Foundation, USA

Ronald Dahl, Aarhus University Hospital NBG, Denmark
Michael Engelgau, US Centers for Disease Control and Prevention, USA
Majid Ezzati, Harvard School of Public Health, USA
Valentin Fuster, World Heart Federation
Pablo Gottret, World Bank
Kei Kawabata, World Bank
Steven Leeder, Australian Health Policy Institute, Australia
Pierre Lefèbvre, International Diabetes Federation
Karen Lock, London School of Hygiene and Tropical Medicine, United Kingdom
James Mann, Human Nutrition and Medicine, University of Otago, New Zealand
Mario Maranhão, World Heart Federation
Stephen Matlin, Global Forum for Health Research, Switzerland
Martin McKee, London School of Hygiene and Tropical Medicine, United Kingdom
Isabel Mortara, International Union Against Cancer
Thomas Pearson, University of Rochester Medical Center, USA

Maryse Pierre-Louis, World Bank

G. N. V. Ramana, World Bank

Anthony Rodgers, University of Auckland, New Zealand

Inés Salas, University of Santiago, Chile

George Schieber, World Bank

Linda Siminerio, International Diabetes Federation

Colin Sindall, Commonwealth Department of Health and Ageing, Australia

Krisela Steyn, Medical Research Council, South Africa

Boyd Swinburn, Deakin University, Australia

Michael Thiede, University of Cape Town, South Africa

Theo Vos, University of Queensland, Australia

Janet Voûte, World Heart Federation

Derek Yach, Yale University School of Medicine, USA

Ping Zhang, US Centers for Disease Control and Prevention, USA

CONTRIBUTORS

CORE CONTRIBUTORS

Dele Abegunde

Robert Beaglehole

Stéfanie Durivage

JoAnne Epping-Jordan

Colin Mathers

Bakuti Shengelia

Kate Strong

Colin Tukuitonga

Nigel Unwin

BACKGROUND CONTRIBUTORS AND REVIEWERS

WHO GENEVA

Dele Abegunde

Denis Aitken

Timothy Armstrong

Robert Beaglehole

Hamadi Benaziza

Ruth Bonita

Victor Boulyjenkov

Guy Carrin

Elenora Cavagnero

Stéfanie Durivage

JoAnne Epping-Jordan

David Evans

Regina Guthold

Irene Hoskins

Sonali Johnson

Jack Jones

Alex Kalache

Nikolai Khaltaev

Chapal Khasnabis

Ivo Kocur

Aku Kwamie

Catherine Le Galès-Camus

Dejan Loncar

Eva Mantzouranis

Silvio Mariotti

Amanda Marlin

Colin Mathers

Paolo Matricardi

Karen McCaffrey

Jane McElligott

Shanthi Mendis

Charlotte Mill

Adepeju Olukoya

Tomoko Ono

Monica Ortegon

Para Pararajasegaram

Poul Erik Petersen

Bruce Pfleger

Thomson Prentice

Serge Resnikoff

Leanne Riley

Gojka Roglic

Caroline Savitzky

Cecilia Sepúlveda

Ruitai Shao

Bakuti Shengelia

Andrew Smith

Ian Smith

Kate Strong

Sameera Suri

Tessa Tan Torres

Kristin Thompson

Thomas Truelsen

Colin Tukuitonga

Andreas Ullrich

Nigel Unwin

Maria Villanueva

Alexi Wright

Hongyi Xu

Ju Yang

WHO REGIONAL AND COUNTRY OFFICES

Mohamed Amri, WHO United Republic of Tanzania Country Office

Alberto Barcelo, WHO Regional Office for the Americas

Robert Burton, WHO China Country Office

Luis Gerardo Castellanos, WHO Brazil Country Office

Lucimar Coser-Cannon, WHO Regional Office for the Americas

Niklas Danielsson, WHO Tonga Country Office

Jill Farrington, WHO Regional Office for Europe

Antonio Filipé Jr, WHO Regional Office for Africa

Gauden Galea, WHO Regional Office for the Western Pacific

Josefa Ippolito-Shepherd, WHO Regional Office for the Americas

Oussama Khatib, WHO Regional Office for the Eastern Mediterranean

Jerzy Leowski, WHO Regional Office for South East Asia

Silvana Luciani, WHO Regional Office for the Americas

Gudjon Magnússon, WHO Regional Office for Europe

Sylvia Robles, WHO Regional Office for the Americas

Aushra Shatchkute, WHO Regional Office for Europe

Marc Suhrcke, WHO Regional Office for Europe

Cristobal Tunon, WHO China Country Office

Cherian Varghese, WHO India Country Office

Mikko Vienonen, WHO Office for the Russian Federation

Wu Yanwei, WHO China Country Office

EXTERNAL CONTRIBUTORS

Marwah Abdalla, Yale University, USA

Josie d'Avernas, Health Promotion Consulting, Canada

Jarbas Barbosa da Silva Júnior, Ministry of Health, Brazil

Ashley Bloomfield, Ministry of Health, New Zealand

Antonio Carlos Cezário, Ministry of Health, Brazil

Deborah Carvalho Malta, Ministry of Health, Brazil

Rhona Hanning, University of Waterloo, Canada

Lenildo de Moura, Ministry of Health, Brazil

Marie DesMeules, Centre for Chronic Disease Prevention and Control, Public Health Agency of Canada

Nancy Dubois, DU B FIT Consulting, Canada

V. Dzerve, National Institute of Cardiology, Latvia

Brodie Ferguson, Stanford University, USA

Igor Glasunov, State Research Centre for Preventive Medicine, Russian Federation

Vilius Grabauskas, Kaunas University of Medicine, Lithuania

Sunjai Gupta, Department of Health, United Kingdom

Lisa Houston, Yale University, USA

Rod Jackson, University of Auckland, New Zealand

Nyoman Kandun, Ministry of Health, Indonesia

J. Klumbiene, Kaunas University of Medicine, Lithuania

T.V. Kamardina, State Research Centre for Preventive Medicine, Russian Federation

Churnrurtai Kanchanachitra, Mahidol University and Thai Health Promotion Foundation, Thailand

A. Kasmel, Estonian Centre for Health Education and Promotion, Estonia

Lingzhi Kong, Ministry of Health, China

Lynne Lane, Food Industry Accord, New Zealand

Tiina Laatikainen, National Public Health Institute, Finland

Otaliba Libânio de Morais, Ministry of Health, Brazil

V. Mohan, Madras Diabetes Research Foundation, India

A. Nissinen, National Public Health Institute, Finland

C.S. Shanthirani, Madras Diabetes Research Foundation, India

Sania Nishtar, Heartfile, Pakistan

Rafael Oganov, State Research Centre for Preventive Medicine, Russian Federation

J. Petkeviciene, Kaunas University of Medicine, Lithuania

Louise Plouffe, Health Canada, Canada

Philip Poole-Wilson, World Heart Federation

M.V. Popovich, State Research Centre for Preventive Medicine, Russian Federation

R.A. Potemkina, State Research Centre for Preventive Medicine, Russian Federation

Enrique Pouget, Yale University, USA

Ritva Prättälä, National Public Health Institute, Finland

I. Pudule, National Institute of Cardiology, Latvia

Natasha Rafter, University of Auckland, New Zealand

A. Ramachandran, Diabetes Research Centre Foundation, India

K. Srinath Reddy, All India Institute of Medical Sciences, India

Anthony Rodgers, University of Auckland, New Zealand

I.M. Solovjeva, State Research Centre for Preventive Medicine, Russian Federation

Krisela Steyn, Medical Research Council, South Africa

Anderson Stanciole, University of York, United Kingdom

M.Viigimaa, Tartu University Hospital, Estonia

Janet Voûte, World Heart Federation

Walter Willett, Harvard School of Public Health, USA

Witold Zatonski, M. Sklodowska-Curie Memorial Cancer Center and Institute of Oncology, Poland

REPORT PRODUCTION

PRODUCTION TEAM
Robert Constandse
Raphaël Crettaz
Steve Ewart
Maryvonne Grisetti
Peter McCarey
Andy Pattison
Thomson Prentice
Reda Sadki
Leo Vita-Finzi

DESIGN
Reda Sadki

LAYOUT
Steve Ewart
Reda Sadki

FIGURES
Steve Ewart
Christophe Grangier

PHOTOGRAPHY
Chris De Bode, Panos Pictures,
   United Kingdom

TECHNICAL EDITING
Leo Vita-Finzi

PROOFREADING
Barbara Campanini

INDEXING
Kathleen Lyle

WHO is grateful to colleagues who supported the *Face to face with chronic disease* project.

Over 40 people with, or affected by, chronic disease were photographed and interviewed by a photojournalist in early 2005. Overall, this set of photographs and stories from five diverse countries demonstrates that chronic diseases are widespread in low and middle income countries and are an underappreciated source of poverty, requiring comprehensive and coordinated responses.

WHO GENEVA
Chris Black
Ivo Kocur
Eva Mantzouranis
Silvio Mariotti
Gopal Prasad Pokharel
Cecilia Sepúlveda
Ruitai Shao
Andrew Smith
Sameera Suri

BRAZIL
Luis Gerardo Castellanos, WHO Brazil
   Country Office
Alberto Barcelo, WHO Regional Office
   for the Americas
Victor Matsudo, Agita São Paulo
   Program, Center of Studies of
   the Physical Fitness Research
   Laboratory, São Caetano do Sul

CHINA
Quingjun Lu, Beijing Tong Ren Eye
   Centre, Tong Ren Hospital, Beijing
You-Lin Qiao, Department of Cancer
   Epidemiology, Cancer Institute,
   Chinese Academy of Medical
   Sciences and Peking Union Medical
   College, Beijing
Gauden Galea, WHO Western Pacific
   Regional Office, Manila
Cristobal Tunon, WHO China Country
   Office, Beijing
Roy Wadia, WHO China Country Office,
   Beijing

INDIA
Pavi Krishnan, Aravind Eye Hospital,
   Madurai
P. Namperumalsamy, Aravind Eye
   Hospital, Madurai
A. Ramachandran, Diabetes Research
   Centre & M.V. Hospital for Diabetes,
   Chennai
N. Murugesan, Diabetes Research
   Centre & M.V. Hospital for Diabetes,
   Chennai

PAKISTAN
Sameer Ashfaq Malik, Heartfile,
   Islamabad
Aamir Javed Khan, Interactive R&D,
   Karachi
Sania Nishtar, Heartfile, Islamabad

UNITED KINGDOM
Sister Teresa Clarke, Saint Joseph's
   Hospice, London
Christina Mason, Saint Joseph's
   Hospice, London
Jo Harkness, International Alliance of
   Patients Organizations, London
Avril Jackson, St Christopher's
   Hospice, London

UNITED REPUBLIC OF TANZANIA
Mohamed Amri, WHO United Republic
   of Tanzania Country Office,
   Dar es Salaam
William Mntenga, WHO United Republic
   of Tanzania Country Office,
   Dar es Salaam

We would like to thank all those people who were willing to tell their story, and have their photo taken, for inclusion in this report and on the WHO web site: http://www.who.int/

Anna Mashishi, WHO United Republic of Tanzania Country Office, Dar es Salaam
Grace E.B. Saguti, Ministry of Health, United Republic of Tanzania, Dar es Salaam
Ahmed Jusabani, Kilimanjaro Stroke Study, Kilimanjaro
Paul Courtright, Kilimanjaro Centre for Community Ophthalmology, Kilimanjaro
Michael Mahande, Kilimanjaro Centre for Community Ophthalmology, Kilimanjaro
Kaushik Ramaiya, International Diabetes Federation, Dar es Salaam
Ramadhan Mongi, International Diabetes Federation, Dar es Salaam
Ferdinand Mugusi, Muhimbili University College of Health Sciences, Dar es Salaam
Edith Ngirwamungu, International Trachoma Initiative, Dar es Salaam,
Twalib A. Ngoma, Ocean Road Cancer Institute, Dar es Salaam

FROM BRAZIL
Maria C. Guimaras Maurho Arruda
Roberto Severino Campos
Vilma Fernandes del Debbio
Milton Paulo Floret Franzolin
Cinthia Mendes Pereira
Noemia Vicente Ribeiro
Luciano dos Santos Rocha Jr
Renilde Fiqueiredo dos Santos
Diego Neri Oliveira e Silva

FROM INDIA
Sharad Arya
Ethi Raj. C.
P.V. Chokkalingam
Kuzhanthiammal
Ravi Mohan
Anandhachari Padma
K. Sridhar Reddy (deceased)
S. Sarswathy
Mana Sekaran
Menaka Seni
A. Vesudevan

FROM PAKISTAN
Muhammed Asgair
Shakeela Begum
Bakht Bibi
Zahida Bibi
Carmilyn Fernandez
Faiz Mohammad
Shakila Nabaz
Ali Raza
Zeenat-Un-Nisa
Muhammed Urfan
Kauser Younis
Ghulam Zohra

FROM THE UNITED REPUBLIC OF TANZANIA
Anita Bulindi
Tkisaeli Oshoseni Masawe
Mariam John
Jonas Justo Kassa (deceased)
Natang'amuraki Koisasi
Eliamulika Lemurtu
Josefu Ramaita Mollel
Mzurisana Mosses
Marystella M. Mtenga
Gerald Ngoroma
Salima Rashidi
Malri Twalib
Maria Saloniki
Ndeshifaya Aron Uronu

FROM THE UNITED KINGDOM
Gillian Crabb
Stephanie Cruickshank
Martin Hession
Melanie Keane
George Smith
Iain Thomas
Lotte Trevatt

Index